THE MEN'S FITNESS
EXERCISE
BIBLE

THE MEN'S FITNESS
EXERCISE BIBLE

101 BEST WORKOUTS TO BUILD MUSCLE, BURN FAT, AND SCULPT YOUR BEST BODY EVER!

By Sean Hyson, C.S.C.S.,
and the Editors of *Men's Fitness*

No book can replace the diagnostic expertise and medical advice of a trusted medical professional. Please be certain to consult a qualified medical professional before beginning an exercise program, particularly if you suffer from any medical condition or have a symptom that may require treatment. You should be in good physical condition and be able to participate in the exercise. When participating in an exercise program, there is the possibility of physical injury, and you do so at your own risk.

Published in the United States by
Galvanized Books,
a division of Galvanized Brands, LLC, New York

Galvanized Books is a trademark of
Galvanized Brands, LLC

DESIGN & ART DIRECTION BY JOSEPH HEROUN
DESIGN BY MIKE SMITH

PHOTOGRAPHY BY BETH BISCHOFF

PHOTO DIRECTION BY JANE SEYMOUR

FOOD PYRAMID ILLUSTRATIONS BY GUYCO

PRINTED IN THE UNITED STATES OF AMERICA ON ACID-FREE PAPER

ISBN 9780989594011

GALVANIZED

Dedication

To all the people who claim they don't have the time or equipment to exercise. Sorry, but you can never use that excuse again.

Acknowledgments

I owe the following people a great debt of gratitude for their work in putting this book together.

Thanks to David Pecker, Chairman and CEO of American Media, Inc.; and to Galvanized Brands, LLC, including David Zinczenko, Stephen Perrine, Joe Heroun, Jon Hammond, and Mike Smith. You trusted me with an enormous project and gave me a golden opportunity.

Thanks also to our amazing photo crew—Beth Bischoff, Antonio Rodriguez, Nate Mumford, Holly Eve Landfield, Jamie Slater, and Jennifer Fleming—whose patience and attention to detail ensured that hundreds of exercises were shot correctly. Props to *Men's Fitness* staffers Emily Luppino, Michael Schletter, and especially to Cat Perry, Shawn Perine, Brian Good, and Jane Seymour for your toughness over many long days and late nights.

To Jim Smith and Ben Bruno, thank you for traveling the many miles required to tech these shoots without hesitation or expectation. Your friendship humbles me. Same goes for Jason Ferruggia, C.J. Murphy, Zach Even-Esh, Joe Stankowski, and all the other fitness pros who contributed workouts and nutrition information. Your real-world expertise is invaluable.

Finally, much love to the readers of *Men's Fitness,* including Kevin and Lynn Hyson, who demanded that I get some exercise back when I was a kid. Now, to their unending surprise, they can't get me to stop.

-Sean Hyson

Contents

Foreword by Dave Zinczenko   xiii

Introduction   1

BEFORE WE BEGIN

1 / The *Men's Fitness* Food Pyramid   5

2 / How to Warm Up   13

FULL BODY WORKOUTS

3 / Full Gym   25

4 / Barbell   49

5 / Dumbbells & Kettlebells   55

6 / Machines   67

7 / Bands   73

8 / Suspension Trainer   79

9 / Medicine Ball   83

10 / Swiss Ball   89

11 / Body Weight   93

BODY PART WORKOUTS

12 / **Arms** 103

13 / **Biceps** 113

14 / **Triceps** 123

15 / **Forearms** 137

16 / **Chest** 145

17 / **Shoulders** 165

18 / **Back** 185

19 / **Legs** 199

20 / **Calves** 215

21 / **Butt** 223

22 / **Abs** 237

23 / **Traps** 253

Contents

UPPER & LOWER BODY WORKOUTS

24 / Upper Body   259

25 / Lower Body   267

CARDIO WORKOUTS

26 / Cardio Machines   273

27 / Body-Weight Cardio   289

28 / Running   297

29 / Boxing & MMA   303

SHORT WORKOUTS

30 / Abs in Under 30 Minutes   315

Foreword
By David Zinczenko,
New York Times best-selling author of *EAT IT TO BEAT IT!* and *THE ABS DIET*

The world's greatest workout is right here in your hands.

That's a heck of a bold statement to make, I admit, because in the end the world's greatest workout is the one that is right for your body, achieves your goals, and fits your time and equipment constraints, and lifestyle. So how can one mere book possibly give you all of that?

Because this book is unlike any other fitness book ever created. Because no matter who you are, what you want, or where you happen to be standing right at this moment, the world's greatest workout–the greatest workout for *you*–is now at your fingertips.

You see, just walking into a gym doesn't guarantee you a great workout. It's a lot like walking into a supermarket. Just because you fill your shopping cart with lots of great food doesn't mean you know how to whip up a great meal. Cook all of those foods too fast, too long, or in the wrong combinations and even the freshest, most expensive ingredients turn into slop.

The same thing happens in the gym: There are dozens of shiny machines and piles of free weights, and literally thousands of things you can do with them to build muscle and burn fat. But simply having access to a lot of equipment doesn't mean you'll know how to craft a great workout–one that will maximize your gains and minimize the time you spend reaching them.

If you've ever been frustrated by fitness plans in the past–or found yourself dropping out because of a lack of results, a lack of time, or because your routine called for equipment that wasn't available on a regular basis, this book is for you. If you want to see progress immediately and feel yourself getting stronger and leaner by the day, this book is for you. If you want to take the gains you've reached and turbocharge them, this book is for you. If you want the perfect workout for the time you have, the equipment you have, and the goals you have, this book is for you.

And most important: If you want total confidence that the workout you're doing is the absolute best possible workout, bar none, this book is for you.

Unlike other exercise books that give you unyielding systems incapable of adapting to time or equipment constraints, or that simply list hundreds of exercises but don't tell you how to meld them into a cohesive workout, this book is different. Like a Swiss Army knife, it's a multifaceted tool that adapts to provide you with the results you want, no matter the circumstances.

As the editorial director of *Men's Fitness,* and the health and wellness editor of ABC News, I've tried just about every exercise plan ever created. I've lifted fast, I've lifted slow; I've lifted heavy, I've lifted light; I've run marathons and I've done wind sprints. (Although I have not, and will not, Zumba.) And I've spent more than 20 years reading studies and theories on building muscle, burning fat, and boosting endurance.

But what makes me excited about this book—what makes it so different from other exercise guides on the market—is that it guarantees you the absolute best workout no matter where you find yourself, what your goals are, or what equipment you have.

Want the ultimate full-body fat-burning workout for the gym? It's in here.

Want the absolute best upper-body workout but have access only to a pair of dumbbells? You're covered.

Want to shred your abs but have nothing but a pair of cross-trainers and a jogging trail? You've got the plan.

Want to build muscle even while you're trapped in a motel room or the world's lamest hotel gym? This book takes every circumstance into consideration and gives you only the best.

I know how good the workouts are in here because I know the team that built them: Sean Hyson, C.S.C.S., has been designing and editing workouts for the readers of *Men's Fitness* and *Muscle & Fitness* for more than 10 years; he may well be the most knowledgeable fitness editor in the business. And I know how good the workouts are because I've done them myself—and they have kicked my ass. I've been astounded by the results!

Now it's time for you to build muscle, burn fat, and get into the greatest shape of your life in record time—all the while knowing that no matter where you are, no matter what equipment you have, the workout you're doing is the absolute best workout for you, with the absolute maximum return on investment.

Get ready to start winning.

David Zinczenko

Introduction

Be your best, wherever, whenever

If you're reading this book, you already appreciate the importance of working out. You know that without a regular training routine you're not going to be your best— and let's face it, being successful at this thing called life means constant striving to become the best you can be.

Of course, when it comes to training—like most everything else in life—sometimes circumstances seem to conspire to keep you from working out. Maybe you'll find yourself on the road without access to a gym or with access to only a really lame one. Or you might be in a situation where the only training equipment at your disposal is a TRX system, bands, or even less. Or maybe you have all the equipment you need but could use a different routine—one that shakes your body out of the complacency that results from sticking with a good thing for too long. You want to be your best, but sometimes that means making the best of a bad situation. Now, thanks to this book, you can always get a great workout—no matter where you are.

Consider this a kind of Rosetta stone for training. No matter what kind of equipment you have (or lack thereof), or your degree of training experience, we've got a workout for you. In fact, we've got 101 of them. Your surroundings will never limit your routine again, with routines for barbells, dumbbells, and even just one dumbbell. You'll find routines that utilize suspension trainers, exercise bands, medicine balls, Swiss balls, or nothing but your body weight alone. And you'll get to handpick from workouts that target the whole body or a program that focuses on body parts individually, along with specific workouts for the upper body and lower body. Plus, we've included routines for every cardio machine imaginable.

With this book, the coast is clear for you to get bigger, stronger, and leaner than ever, sculpting the body you've always wanted, regardless of your resources.

Now, like most everything, this book has an upside and a downside. On the upside, you now have a resource that covers all your workout needs under every conceivable circumstance. The question "What kind of workout should I do?" has been answered forever. On the downside, you have no more excuses. You can't skip sessions because you're on the road and your hotel has a crappy, antiquated, little gym or no gym at all. Hell, you don't even have an excuse to skip a workout if you're lost in the arctic tundra (see page 100)! You also can no longer say that you don't have time to train, because some of these workouts require less time than an average water-cooler conversation (there's a dedicated section of short workouts ranging from 30 minutes down to only four).

This body-carving tome will fast-track your gains and teach you how to upgrade your current routine easily, with an incredible array of body-challenging routines. One hundred one options is a surefire plateau buster.

Nearly as diverse as the workouts within these pages are the fitness experts we've recruited to design them, providing you with a wealth of authoritative information that has stood the test of thousands of training clients.

Yet because training is only half the equation of physique transformation, we've also got your nutrition needs covered. Our newly erected *Men's Fitness* Food Pyramid provides you with a foundation for building muscle while losing fat, employing the simplest calculations and menu plan.

So, as of right now, you officially have no more limitations to your training—at least when it comes to location, time, and equipment. And, for better or worse, that also means no more excuses. With this book, the world becomes your gym—one that's open 24/7, 365 days— with everything you need to build loads of quality muscle. Take advantage of your membership today and you're guaranteed to look and feel your best for a lifetime to come.

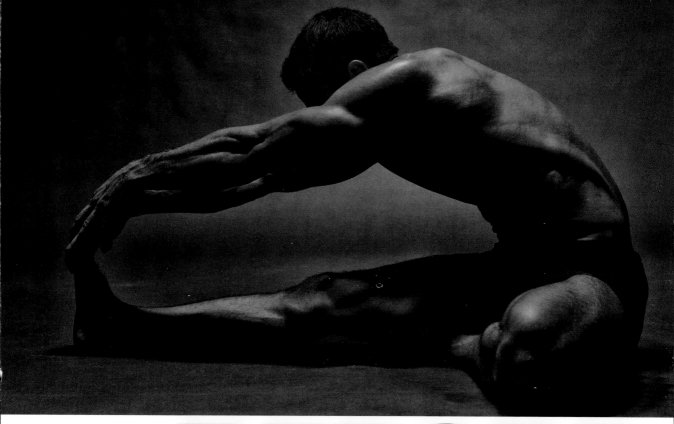

BEFORE
WE BEGIN

01 THE *MEN'S FITNESS* FOOD PYRAMID

Remember the USDA Food Pyramid? The one that was posted by the lunch line in your grade school cafeteria and taught in health class? The government's official position on how you should eat to be fit and healthy included recommendations to consume up to 11 servings of pasta, bread, and crackers per day; limit meat and eggs to three servings; and count potatoes as a vegetable.

Yeah, don't eat like that.

The Food Pyramid was so misleading and inaccurate that in 2011 it was replaced with the USDA's MyPlate, an improved but still flawed approach to fighting obesity. To be fair, the government's nutrition advice is aimed at the average American who desires to be in only average shape (read: not obese). As we assume you picked up this book to be bigger, stronger, more ripped, and healthier than that, you need an entirely different approach.

To that end, we've created the *Men's Fitness* Food Pyramid–an easy visual guide to eating for physique enhancement, performance, and optimal health. See how the pyramid works below and then use it to build a better body.

HIT YOUR NUMBERS

As a physique-conscious eater, you need to think in terms of macronutrients as well as calories. Every food you eat gets counted toward a total target amount (in grams) of protein, carbs, and fat, which you can determine by multiplying the numbers in the *Men's Fitness* Food Pyramid by your body weight in pounds. Hit these numbers and you'll hit your goals.

With that said, your nutrition doesn't need to be as precise as target coordinates for a missile attack. You'll do just fine eyeballing portions of protein, carbs, and fat (which we'll show you how to do) and keeping a general tally.

MAKE ADJUSTMENTS AS NECESSARY

The calorie and macronutrient recommendations here are just a starting point. Every trainee needs to find the proper amounts for his own body. If you're not losing weight, reduce your carbs gradually, and try experimenting with bumping up your protein and fat intake a bit. If you feel as if you can't gain weight, you can add more carbs and even more fat, which will increase your calories sharply. For any formulation you make, give it at least a week to take effect before you make any changes.

PROTEIN

With protein being the main component of muscle tissue, your intake of it must remain high no matter your goal. To make size gains, you need at least one gram of protein per pound of your body weight to support optimal growth. When dieting, you must create a caloric deficit–but that can cause muscle loss if you end up cutting protein to do it. That's why we increase protein intake and decrease starchy carbs. To get lean, you may

The *Men's Fitness* Food Pyramid was created with cooperation from the *Men's Fitness* Nutrition Advisory Board. It includes John Meadows, C.S.S.N.; Nate Miyaki, C.S.S.N.; Chris Mohr, Ph.D.; and Shelby Starnes.

FAT LOSS
Eat like this to lose fat

FAT
0.4 GRAMS PER POUND
OF BODY WEIGHT

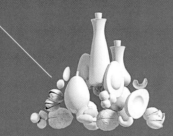

PROTEIN
1-1.5 GRAMS PER POUND

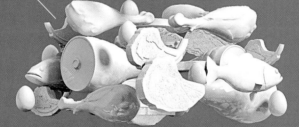

CARBS
1 GRAM PER POUND

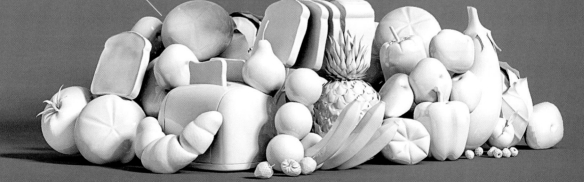

MUSCLE GAIN
Eat like this to put on muscle

CALORIES
14–18 PER POUND

FAT
0.4 GRAMS PER POUND
OF BODY WEIGHT

PROTEIN
1–1.5 GRAMS PER POUND

CARBS
2 GRAMS PER POUND

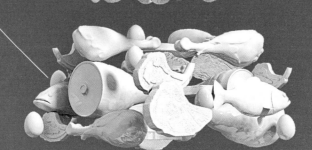

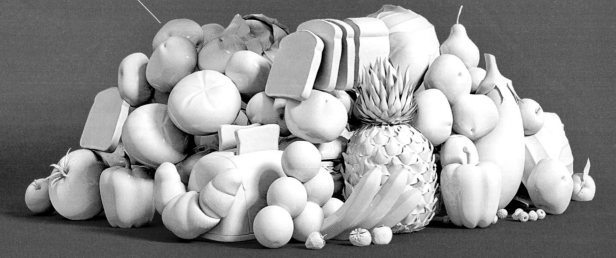

increase your protein to as many as 1.5 grams per pound of body weight; but start lower and increase gradually as you reduce your calories slowly. If you feel like you're not recovering from training or you're losing muscle, up the protein fast.

The best protein sources are eggs, chicken, fish, lean beef, turkey, quinoa (for vegetarians), and protein powder. A three-ounce portion of lean meat or fish is about the size and thickness of the palm of your hand and contains 20-25 grams of protein, five grams of fat or fewer, and zero carbs.

CARBS

All carbohydrates break down into glucose, raising your blood sugar levels faster than any other nutrient. As a result, the pancreas releases insulin to remove surplus sugar from the bloodstream and maintain normal levels. Research, including a study at the University of Washington School of Medicine, has found that exercise–particularly strength training–increases insulin sensitivity in the muscles. So if you've just worked out, more of the carbs you eat afterward will be carried by insulin directly to your muscles for replenishment. (Incidentally, this goes for protein too, which is why it's helpful to consume a mixture of protein and carbs after training–we'll discuss this more later.) On the other hand, if you've been sitting on the couch watching football, those carbs will just get stored around your waist.

For this reason, we recommend that most of your carbs come before, during, and shortly after training. It also means that you need to eat fewer carbs when you want to get lean–you need to keep insulin levels low. "If someone is in fat-loss mode," says John Meadows, C.S.S.N., a nutrition coach and national-level bodybuilder, "I like to limit carbs to pre-, intra-, and post-workout meals, when they'll go where you want them"–that is, to muscle tissue. For muscle gain, Meadows prefers to add carbs (shakes included) to meals around training time first, before adding them to other meals.

Carb foods include potatoes, sweet potatoes, rice, oats, fruits, and vegetables. Fruits should be consumed in their whole-food form and limited to two or three pieces daily (excess fructose, the sugar in fruit, is stored as fat). Green vegetables can be eaten steadily regardless of the goal. Eat one gram of carbohydrate per pound of your body weight when dieting and two grams per pound when you want to put on muscle.

A fist-size portion of cooked rice or potatoes is about one cup and gives you 40-45 grams of carbs and negligible protein and fat.

FAT

"We need to provide a baseline level of good fats for hormone production," says Nate Miyaki, C.S.S.N., a nutrition consultant and bodybuilder in San Francisco, CA. Fat, particularly the much-maligned saturated kind, helps in the creation of testosterone, which does everything from getting you big and lean to keeping your "little friend" ready to say hello. Contrary to popular opinion, when dieting, you don't need to drop your fat intake much, if at all; fat loss comes fastest when carbohydrate intake is reduced. Plus, fat is satiating as well as a good source of energy.

Most of your fats should come by way of your protein foods, but avocados, nuts, seeds, and a small amount of oil like coconut and olive oil can be included as well. Aim for 0.4 grams per pound of your body weight daily to start. One tablespoon of any oil is about 15 grams of fat, and one cup of almonds or peanuts has 70 grams of fat. Two tablespoons of nut butter is about the length of your thumb and contains 15-20 grams of fat.

WORKOUT NUTRITION

Research hasn't yet clarified the optimal amount of protein or carbs you should eat around workouts for the maximum benefit. But it is clear that some is better than none, and the presence of both is crucial. A 2006 study in the *European Journal of Applied Physiology* gave male subjects one of the following to consume after weight training: a 6 percent carbohydrate solution, six grams of amino acids (components of protein), a combination of both, or a placebo. Those drinking the carb-and-aminos shake experienced greater muscle gains than any of the other groups, which the researchers presumed was because the concoction did the most to reduce muscle protein breakdown after training.

Meadows recommends taking in 25-50 grams of protein, 25-35 grams of carbs, and 10 grams of fat before training. Afterward, consume another 20-40 grams of protein and 40-80 grams of carbs—you can begin chugging this shake during the workout as well to limit muscle breakdown even further, though this may not be necessary and could upset your stomach. We like to make shakes with whey isolate or hydrolysate as the protein source, and Vitargo or highly branched cyclic dextrin for carbs.

If powders and shakes aren't in your budget, Miyaki says you can go old-school and eat fruit pre- and post-workout. One or two pieces should provide enough carbs to halt muscle breakdown. And a lean three-ounce slice of protein to accompany it is fine.

A PERFECT DAY

How to plan your eating to achieve your goals

Let's say you're a

180

POUND MAN who wants to lose his gut.

You could start your diet eating about

2,100

CALORIES DAILY

(180 x 12)

consisting of

180g

PROTEIN,

180g

CARBS,

and

70g

FAT.

HERE'S A LOW-STRESS EATING PLAN TO FIT THIS GUY'S BUSY SCHEDULE.

BREAKFAST

8 oz black coffee

3 scrambled eggs

1/3 cup unsweetened oatmeal
with cinnamon

POST-WORKOUT

25g whey protein

1 banana

LUNCH

3 oz grilled salmon

Large raw salad w/ 2 tbsp
olive oil and vinegar

1 cup sweet potato or white potato (cooked)

DINNER

6 oz baked chicken breast

1 cup jasmine rice or potato (cooked)

Steamed broccoli

SNACK

Meal-replacement shake with
50g protein, 25g carbs, 5g fat

DESSERT

2 tbsp almond butter mixed with
one scoop chocolate casein protein
and water (to make a pudding)

02 HOW TO WARM UP

We'll keep this brief. When you're eager to work out, the last thing you want to do is slow your roll with a long warmup that has you flopping around the floor like a fish, draining your momentum. If you passed fifth grade P.E., you've already had it drilled into you that warming up is crucial and not to be skipped, so we'll spare you the speech about howimportant it is. Instead of lecturing, we'll give you some warmup options that get you sweating and ready to perform any of the workouts that follow, but also fit into the time you have and your level of patience—whatever the case may be. Most important is that you don't start lifting heavy weights, jumping, or running totally cold, which common sense should tell you is an injury waiting to happen.

OPTION 1 **THE BEST WARMUP**

If you have at least an hour in which to train, or a history of injuries that could otherwise impede your ability to train safely, your warmup should begin with foam rolling and include a wide array of dynamic exercises and static stretches.

A) If you've tried a foam roller after a tough workout, you were instantly aware of its ability to help relieve muscle aches and soreness. It also provides an easy way to start getting warmed up, as it promotes blood flow. Rest your muscles on the roller (a tennis ball, softball, or lacrosse ball work, too) and roll them out for about 30 seconds each. When you find a tender spot, hold the position until you feel it begin to release (or for as long as you can stand it). Pay extra attention to the hips, glutes, outer and inner thighs, lower back, calves, and lats. You can repeat the rolling after your workout as well if you like, as this may enhance recovery.

B) Perform some light activity that elevates your heart rate and makes you feel warm (though not necessarily fuzzy). This could be a set of 30 jumping jacks, a five-minute walk on the treadmill (set to a slight incline), or a minute or two of jumping rope. Other cardio machines like a stationary bike or an elliptical machine can also get your blood flowing.

C) Now you'll begin what's often called a dynamic warmup. In addition to encouraging further blood flow and higher body temperature, dynamic exercises take your muscles through the ranges of motion you'll use in your workout, preparing you to get into those positions safely. There are endless options, but try this routine.

1 SHOULDER OVER AND BACK

PERFORM 15 REPS

Hold a band, dowel, yardstick, or light bar in front of your hips with hands outside shoulder width. Keeping your elbows straight, raise your arms overhead and behind your body as far as you can. Bring them back in front of you again. Continue going over and back and gradually narrow your grip as you feel your shoulders loosen up.

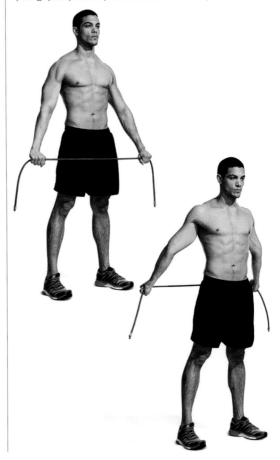

2 HIP HINGE

PERFORM 15 REPS

Place your hands on your hips and stand with feet hip width. Push your hips back, bending your knees only as needed, until you feel a stretch in your hamstrings. Squeeze your glutes as you forcefully push your hips forward again to stand up straight.

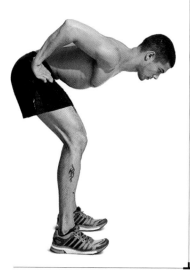

3 OVERHEAD SQUAT

PERFORM 10 REPS

Hold a band, dowel, yardstick, or light bar overhead with hands outside shoulder width. Stand with feet shoulder width and toes turned out slightly. Bend your hips back and squat as low as you can without letting your tailbone tuck under. Keep the object you're holding above and slightly behind your head the whole time—don't let it drift in front of you.

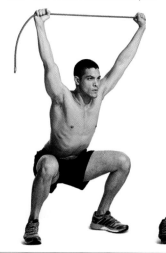

4 SIDE LUNGE

PERFORM 10 REPS ON EACH LEG

Stand with feet hip width and step out to your left. Lower your body until your left knee is bent 90 degrees, or until you feel a stretch in the right side of your groin, but keep your right leg straight. Repeat on the right side.

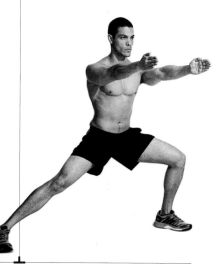

5 BENTOVER YTW

PERFORM 8 REPS OF EACH

Stand with feet shoulder width and bend your hips back, keeping your lower back flat, until your torso is about 45 degrees to the floor. Let your arms hang. Now squeeze your shoulder blades together and raise your arms up and out to your sides about 45 degrees to form a Y shape. Lower them and then raise them out to your sides 90 degrees to form a T. Lower and then raise them out to your sides, but bend your elbows 90 degrees to form a W.

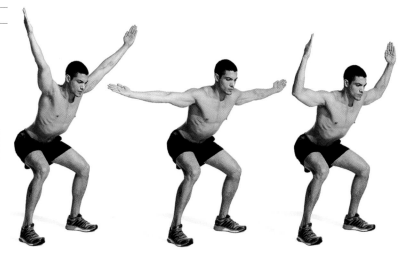

6 CAT/CAMEL

PERFORM 10 REPS

Kneel on the floor with knees under your hips and hands beneath your shoulders. Arch your back so your chest rises—you should look like a cat stretching. Now round your entire back so it looks like a camel's hump.

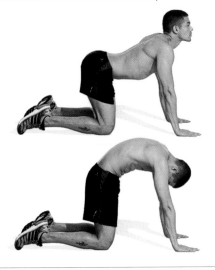

7 BIRD DOG

PERFORM 10 REPS ON EACH SIDE

From the kneeling position, extend your left hand out in front of you. Simultaneously kick your right leg back straight, bracing your core and squeezing your glutes as you do so. Hold for a moment and then switch legs.

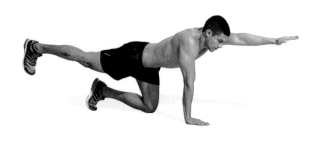

8 HIP CIRCLE

MAKE 10 CLOCKWISE CIRCLES AND THEN SWITCH LEGS; REPEAT ON BOTH LEGS IN THE COUNTERCLOCKWISE DIRECTION

From the kneeling position, raise your right knee off the floor and make circles with it, opening your hip as much as possible on each revolution. Keep your shoulders square to the floor.

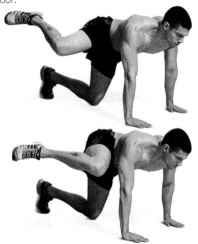

9 GROINER

PERFORM 10 REPS ON EACH SIDE

Get into pushup position with your hands shoulder width, feet close together, and body in a straight line. Jump your left foot forward and land it to the outside of your left hand. Let your hips sink a bit to feel the stretch and then reverse it—jump your left foot back while the right one comes up to your right hand.

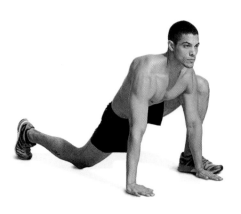

D) At this point, it's wise to statically stretch muscles that you know to be chronically tight. For most people, the hips, glutes, and lats are bound up due to many hours sitting at desks in front of computers, but stretch whatever areas you feel need it most. Hold each stretch for 30 seconds and repeat for three sets on each side. The following are some suggestions.

LAT STRETCH

Grasp a sturdy upright object with your left hand, thumb facing up, and bend your hips back until your torso and arm are in line and you feel a stretch in your lat. Move gently from side to side so you stretch the entire muscle.

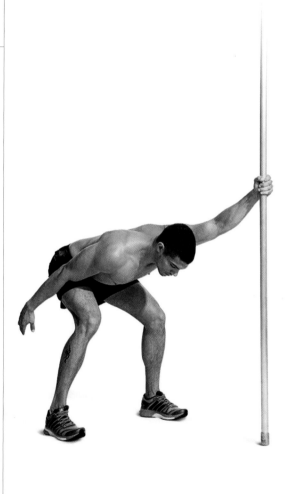

HIP FLEXOR STRETCH

Get into lunge position on the floor with your right leg back. Place your hands on your hips and push your hips forward until you feel a stretch in your right hip. Squeeze your glutes on your right side. For a more intense stretch, reach your right arm overhead and lean back slightly while keeping your hips forward. Another progression is to reach back and grasp the outside of your rear foot and gently pull it off the floor. You'll feel the stretch go into the top of your thigh.

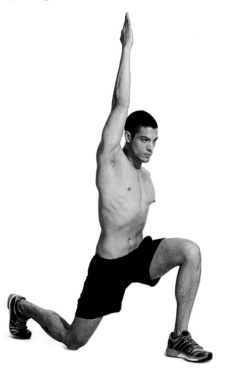

PEC STRETCH

Place the meat of your right forearm against a sturdy upright object (a doorframe is perfect) and bend your elbow 90 degrees. Gently lean forward so you feel a stretch on your pec.

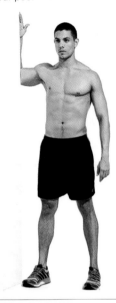

PIRIFORMIS STRETCH

Sit on a bench and cross your left leg over your right knee, bending your left knee 90 degrees. Gently push your left knee down so you feel a stretch on the outside of your left glutes.

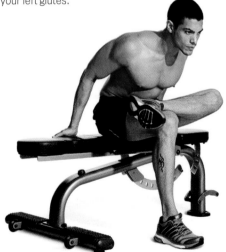

CALF STRETCH

Place your hands against a wall and stagger your feet so one is close to the wall and your rear leg is straight. Both feet face forward and your rear leg should be aligned with your upper body. Lean forward until you feel your calf stretch on your trailing leg.

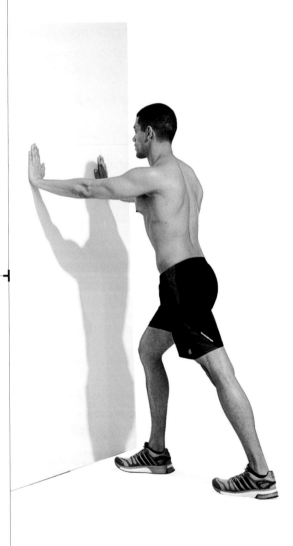

OPTION 2
THE MEATHEAD'S WARMUP

Most guys come into the gym and grasp the bar or a pair of dumbbells and do a light set of 15-20 reps. Then they go a little heavier and cut the reps down a bit. They'll do one more set and, now that they're sweating, figure they're ready to go.

While this is hardly the best way to prep your body, it does serve the purpose most of the time, assuming you're not training too heavy. But take it a little slower and more deliberately, and you've got a more decent warmup routine for when you're doing one of our lifting workouts and need to get done in a hurry.

Here's how to warm up for a heavy strength workout that begins with a barbell exercise. More accurately, this is called "working up" in powerlifting circles, because the goal is to gradually work your way up to using the heaviest weights possible. You start with the empty bar and perform 10-15 reps with perfect form and then add weight in moderate increments until you're at the maximum load you plan to lift on the exercise.

Here's how it might look for a guy working up to a 275-pound squat for five reps:

WEIGHT	Bar	95	135	175	215	255	275
REPS	10	8	5	5	5	5	5
							WORK SET

There's no exact formula for how to do this, so the weights and reps above aren't mandatory, but the idea is to start very light, pump some blood into the working muscles and lubricate the joints, and then add weight steadily until you comfortably arrive at the heaviest load you can use for the target reps. The reps on these work-up sets are kept low (after the first set or two) because you need to conserve energy for the main effort, the work set. These sets also serve to reinforce good technique, so the form on the exercise is fresh in your mind and the body is in its groove to do it properly when you get to a challenging load.

How long should you rest between sets? Since work-up sets aren't as taxing as your main work sets, you shouldn't need to rest long. A minute or so will be fine for most until you get up to heavy weights, at which time you can rest longer.

There are a few tricks you can employ to make this process even more effective and make your top set even heavier, or at least feel easier. Try doing your last work-up set a little heavier than the main set, but only for one or two reps, so it's not too strenuous. Then back down to the weight you intend to use for the work set.

For instance, if you're going to perform a squat with 275 for five, your last four sets could look like this:

WEIGHT	215	255	300	275
REPS	5	3	1	5
			HEAVIER WARMUP	WORK SET

In other words, you gradually work up to an even heavier weight, reducing your reps to minimize fatigue, and then go back down to 275. The set with 300 might be way more than you can handle for five reps, but done for only one, it will feel relatively easy. By comparison, 275 will feel much easier when it's done afterward. Obviously, this won't work on super-heavy sets when your target reps are in the 1-3 range, but it's great when they're between 4 and 8.

Another trick, which we learned from Jason Ferruggia, a strength coach in Los Angeles, CA, is to back the weight down for a set before you reach your target. This works well if you're trying to hit a new max (one rep), which can be very intimidating. The weight tends to feel very heavy at around 90 percent of your max, and it can dissuade you from going any heavier. By going a bit lighter for a set and then working your way back up, you give your nervous system more time to adapt. The weight feels lighter, so you feel more confident, and the rest of the way up to your max weight goes smoother.

Say you're trying to bench press 315 for the first time. Your last few sets could develop like this:

						BACK DOWN		NEW MAX
WEIGHT	135	175	215	245	275	255	285	315
REPS	5	5	3	3	1	1	1	1
					FELT HARD		BACK UP	

To be clear, working up is not optional. Because it can be time consuming, if you have time for only one kind of warmup, this should be it. But we strongly suggest that, whenever possible, you employ one of the other options we list here beforehand.

Incidentally, working up applies to training with kettlebells/dumbbells, a suspension trainer, and bands as well. Start with light resistance, gradually tapering your reps as you up the intensity.

OPTION 3
THE PRACTICAL WARMUP

As the name implies, this routine is for when you have time to warm up, but not enough to do everything listed in Option 1. In this case, you need to get a good sweat going and prepare your muscles and joints to move while doing the bare essentials.

According to Ben Bruno, a celebrity trainer at Rise Movement in West Hollywood, CA, you should hit a cardio machine for five minutes followed by these stretches. "Do toe-touch squats and sumo squat holds (both of which are explained below) to improve mobility," Bruno says.

TOE-TOUCH SQUAT

Stand with feet shoulder width and toes turned slightly out. Reach down to touch your toes with legs extended and then bend your hips back to squat down, keeping your lower back in its natural arch. Now reach your hands overhead and come up.

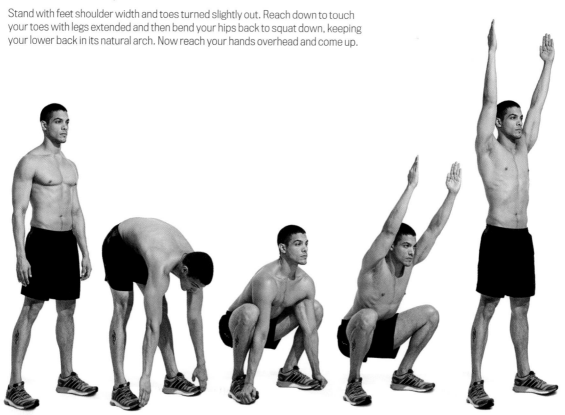

SUMO SQUAT HOLD

Stand with feet shoulder width and toes turned slightly out. Bend your hips back and squat down, keeping your lower back flat and reaching your hands to your toes in the bottom position. Hold the position for a few seconds and then use your elbows to push your knees farther apart so you can sink deeper into the squat.

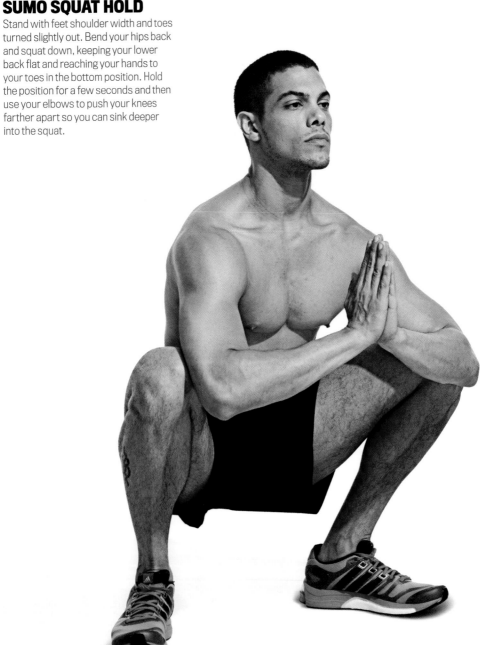

DID WE SAY THIS WOULD BE BRIEF?

In a nutshell, that's all you need to know about warming up. Note that even if you're doing a lower-body workout, it's smart to include some upper-body warmup moves because the entire body is connected. Tightness or coldness in the upper torso can lead to injury when working the legs, and vice versa; so while you may abbreviate or recombine the warmup moves listed here, don't ignore whole muscle areas just because you're not training them that day. For the cardio routines beginning in chapter 26, you don't need to do any more warming up than what is already built into the workouts.

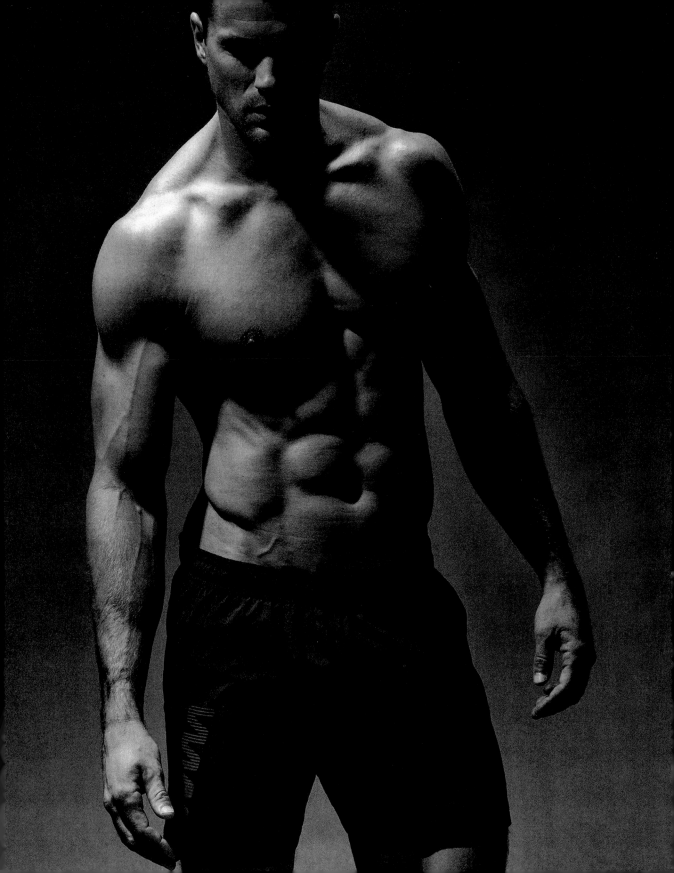

FULL BODY WORKOUTS

03

FULL GYM

We all love to bitch about our gyms. They don't have enough benches, the machines are always broken, and so on. It's only when we're forced to train at home or in a hotel that we realize what a luxury even the most average commercial fitness center is.

If you're lucky enough to have a membership to a training facility, this chapter is for you. Or, if you've put together a well-stocked home gym, this is where you should start as well. While it may not be the fitness paradise you crave, it almost certainly has all the tools you need to build a great body. The workouts that follow will show you how to take advantage of them.

We're assuming your gym has barbells, dumbbells, a powerrack, adjustable benches, cables, Swiss balls, and pullup bars. With that much inventory, you can easily complete the various options of workouts we outline for you. These include three distinct routines for gaining muscle, two for losing fat, and two for body recomposition—workouts that hit the magical combination of both muscle gain and fat loss to reshape your physique with minimal change in body weight.

THE BEST BODY-RECOMPOSITION WORKOUT [option A]

WORKOUT #1   BY JOE DOWDELL, C.S.C.S.

We can't overstate the awesomeness of German engineering. The land that brought us jet planes, the Mercedes, and Heidi Klum also introduced perhaps the best method of body recomposition known to the fitness industry— that is, a timeless strategy to gain muscle and lose body fat simultaneously. *Achtung!*

HOW IT WORKS Hala Rambie, a scientist who defected to West Germany during the Cold War, found that fat loss could be accelerated by raising levels of blood lactate—an energy substrate. More lactate corresponds to greater release of growth hormone, which tells your body to grow muscle and burn flab.

The best way to raise lactate quickly is to pair upper- and lower-body exercises, or opposing movements, for reps in the 8–15 range. The sweet spot for sets is three, and rest periods are restricted to 30–60 seconds. This approach has since become known as German Body Comp.

DIRECTIONS Alternate sets of "A" and "B" exercises. So you'll do a set of A, rest, then a set of B, rest again, and so on for all the prescribed sets. The remaining exercises are done as straight sets.

To increase the intensity, decrease your rest between sets by 15 seconds every two weeks. Start by resting 60 seconds for the first two weeks. Then in Weeks 3 and 4, rest 45 seconds, and so on.

1A DEADLIFT

SETS: 3 REPS: 8-10 TEMPO*: 4010 REST: 60 SEC.

Stand with your feet hip width. Bend your hips back to reach down and grasp the bar, hands just outside your knees. Keeping your lower back in its natural arch, drive your heels into the floor and pull the bar up along your shins until you're standing with hips fully extended and the bar is in front of your thighs.

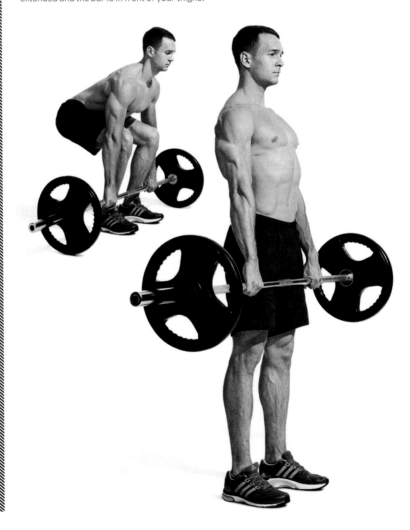

1B 1¼ NEUTRAL-GRIP DUMBBELL BENCH PRESS

SETS: 3 REPS: 8-10 TEMPO: 3020 REST: 60 SEC.

Lie back on a flat bench with a dumbbell in each hand. Turn your wrists so your palms face each other. Press the weights over your chest and then lower back down. Come back up one quarter of the way, and then down again. Now press up to lockout once more. That's one rep. Take three seconds to lower the weights down from the lockout position, and two seconds when pressing to lockout.

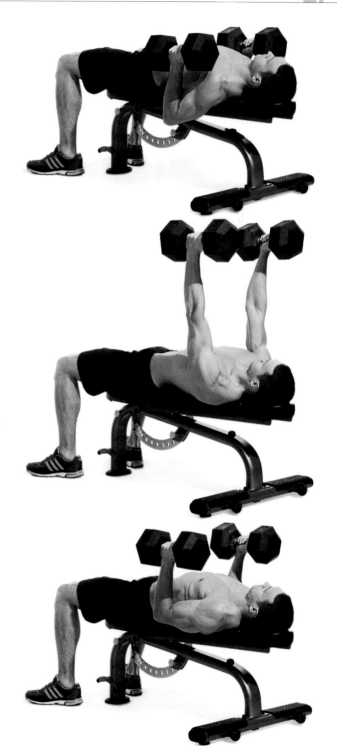

*TEMPO Each exercise is assigned a tempo.

3110

FIRST DIGIT	SECOND DIGIT	THIRD DIGIT	FOURTH DIGIT
seconds you should take to lower the weight	seconds you should pause in the bottom position	applies to the lifting portion of the exercise	the length of the pause in the end position

(A "0" indicates no time–simply move on to the next digit.) For example, a front squat with a tempo of 3110 would be done like so: Take three seconds to lower yourself into the squat. Pause for one second at the bottom. Take one second to come back up to standing, and then go right back into the descent.

2A BULGARIAN SPLIT SQUAT

SETS: 3 REPS: 8-10 (EACH SIDE)
TEMPO: 3110 REST: 60 SEC.

Stand lunge-length in front of a bench. Hold a dumbbell in each hand and rest the top of your left foot on the bench behind you. Lower your body until your rear knee nearly touches the floor and your front thigh is parallel to the floor.

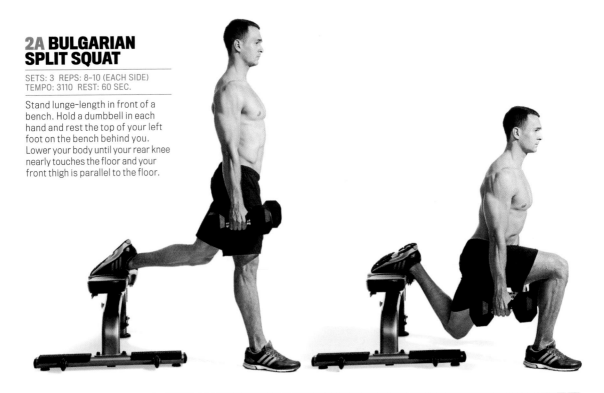

2B INVERTED ROW

SETS: 3 REPS: 10-12 TEMPO: 2011
REST: 60 SEC.

Set a barbell in a power rack (or use a Smith machine) at about hip height. Lie underneath it and grasp it with hands about shoulder-width apart. Hang from the bar so your body forms a straight line. Squeeze your shoulder blades together and pull yourself up until your back is fully contracted.

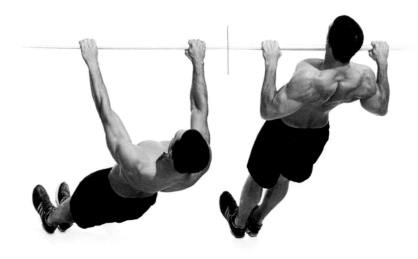

3A DIP

SETS: 3 REPS: 10–12 TEMPO: 3110 REST: 60 SEC.

Suspend yourself over the bars of a dip station and lower your body until your upper arms are parallel to the floor.

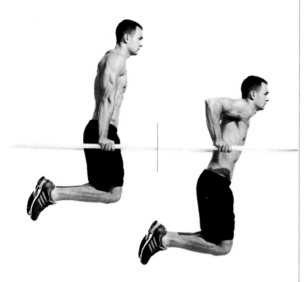

3B SEATED INCLINE DUMBBELL CURL

SETS: 3 REPS: 10–12 TEMPO: 4010 REST: 60 SEC.

Set an adjustable bench between 45 and 60 degrees and sit back against it with a dumbbell in each hand. Curl the weights to shoulder height without allowing your elbows to drift in front of your shoulders.

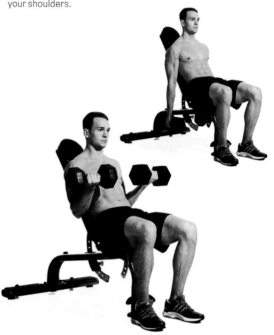

4 SWISS BALL ROLLOUT

SETS: 3 REPS: 10–15 TEMPO: 2020 REST: 60 SEC.

Kneel on the floor and rest your forearms on a Swiss ball. Keeping your core braced, roll the ball forward so your arms are extended. Stop before your lower back begins to sag. Roll yourself back.

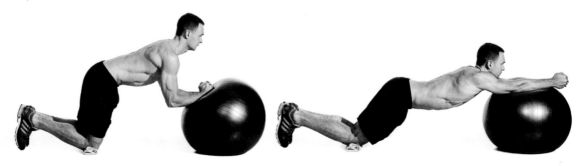

THE BEST BODY-RECOMPOSITION
WORKOUT [option B]

WORKOUT #2   BY JOE DOWDELL, C.S.C.S.

Use this routine just as you did the previous one–Body-Recomposition Option A. It's another example of German Body Comp training and can be done in conjunction with Option A. If you choose to do the two workouts for a few weeks, alternate them for three sessions per week, resting a day between workouts (and then two days afterward before repeating).

1A FRONT SQUAT

SETS: 3 REPS: 8-10 TEMPO: 3110 REST: 60 SEC.

Set a barbell on a power rack at about shoulder height. Grasp the bar with hands at shoulder width and raise your elbows until your upper arms are parallel to the floor. Take the bar out of the rack and let it rest on your fingertips—as long as your elbows stay up, you'll be able to balance the bar. Step back and set your feet at shoulder width with toes turned out slightly. Squat as low as you can without losing the arch in your lower back.

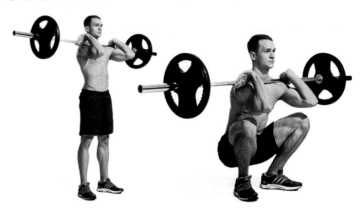

1B NEUTRAL-GRIP CHINUP

SETS: 3 REPS: 8-10 TEMPO: 4010
REST: 60 SEC.

Use a chinup bar that has handles so you can grasp it with your palms facing each other (if you have only a straight bar, hook a V-grip cable handle over it, or use a suspension trainer as shown). Hang from the handles and then pull yourself up until your chin is over them.

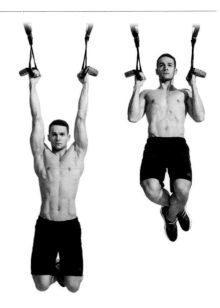

2A ROMANIAN DEADLIFT

SETS: 3 REPS: 8–10 TEMPO: 3110
REST: 60 SEC.

Hold a barbell with a shoulder-width
grip and stand with feet hip width.
Bend your hips back as far as you
can. Allow your knees to bend as
needed while you lower the bar
along your shins until you feel a
stretch in your hamstrings. Keep
your lower back arched throughout.

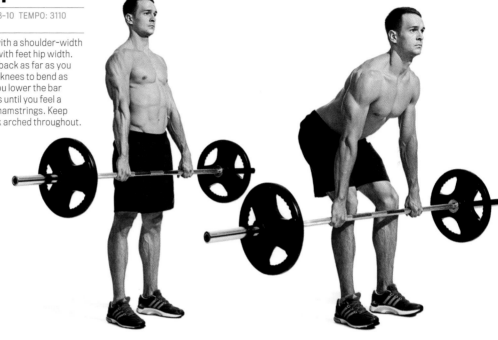

2B INCLINE NEUTRAL-GRIP BENCH PRESS

SETS: 3 REPS: 10–12 TEMPO: 3110 REST: 60 SEC.

Set an adjustable bench to a 30- to 45-degree angle and lie back
on it with a dumbbell in each hand. Turn your wrists so your palms
face each other. Press the weights straight over your chest.

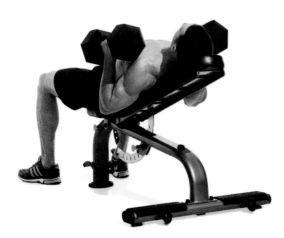
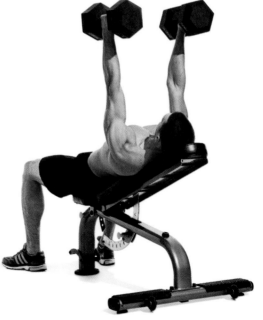

3A SEATED ZOTTMAN CURL

SETS: 3 REPS: 10–12 TEMPO: 3020
REST: 60 SEC.

Hold a dumbbell in each hand and sit down on a bench with a back rest, or raise the back of an adjustable bench to vertical. Curl the weights up and then rotate your wrists so your palms face the floor. Slowly lower your arms back to the starting position.

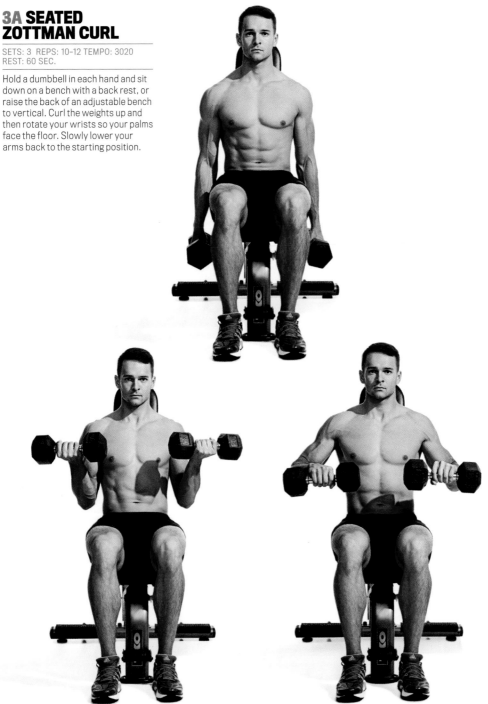

3B DECLINE EZ-BAR TRICEPS EXTENSION

SETS: 3 REPS: 10-12 TEMPO: 4010 REST: 60 SEC.

Set an adjustable bench to a slight decline and lie back against it holding an EZ-curl bar with an overhand, shoulder-width grip. Press the bar overhead and then let your upper arms drift back so they're at an angle to your torso. Bend your elbows so you lower the bar behind your head. Keeping your upper arms stationary, extend your elbows to lock the bar out.

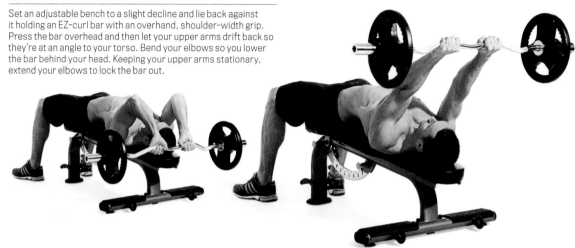

4 HALF-KNEELING CABLE CHOP

SETS: 3 REPS: 8-10 (EACH SIDE)
TEMPO: 3010 REST: 60 SEC.

Attach a rope handle to the top pulley of a cable station. Get into a lunge position, resting your left knee on the floor. Pull the cable diagonally downward to your left side.

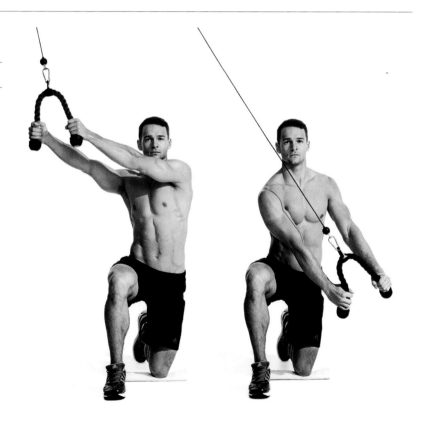

THE BEST FULL-BODY
MUSCLE WORKOUT [option A]

WORKOUT #3   BY SEAN HYSON, C.S.C.S.

Full-body workouts sound like they would take a long time. But when you boil down the exercises you need to perform in order to cover every area, there are only three you need to be concerned with—a push, a pull, and a squat. This is the ultimate in minimalism and works superbly for beginners or people who are short on time.

HOW IT WORKS Any kind of pressing exercise will train your chest, shoulders, and triceps. Any pulling movement (a row or chinup variation) recruits your back, rear delts, biceps, and forearms. Squatting movements (and deadlifts, which aren't quite a squat but require all the same muscles) take care of the quads, hamstrings, and glutes. Even your calves get some stimulation as they help to stabilize your squat. Your abs, of course, get worked on all these movement patterns, provided they're done with free weights rather than machines, and work to brace your spine throughout.

The workout at right contains everything you need to put on size fast—a squat, press, and pullup—done with heavy weights, and you should be able to wrap it up within 45 minutes.

DIRECTIONS Complete all five sets for the squat and then perform the overhead press and weighted pullup in alternating fashion. That is, complete a set of the press, rest, then do a set of the pullup, rest again, and repeat until you've finished all five sets for each.

1 SQUAT

SETS: 5 REPS: 5 REST: 120 SEC.

Set up in a squat rack or cage. Grasp the bar as far apart as is comfortable and step under it. Squeeze your shoulder blades together and nudge the bar out of the rack. Step back and stand with your feet shoulder width and your toes turned slightly outward. Take a deep breath and bend your hips back and then bend your knees to lower your body as far as you can without losing the arch in your lower back. Push your knees outward as you descend. Extend your hips to come back up, continuing to push your knees outward.

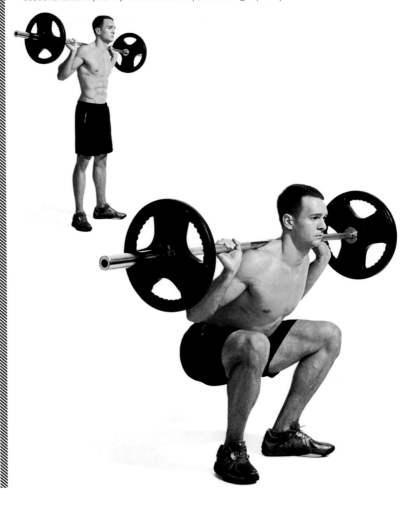

2A OVERHEAD PRESS

SETS: 5 REPS: 5 REST: 60 SEC.

Set the bar up in a squat rack or cage and grasp it just outside shoulder width. Take the bar off the rack and hold it at shoulder level with your forearms perpendicular to the floor. Squeeze the bar and brace your abs. Press the bar overhead, pushing your head forward and shrugging your traps as the bar passes your face.

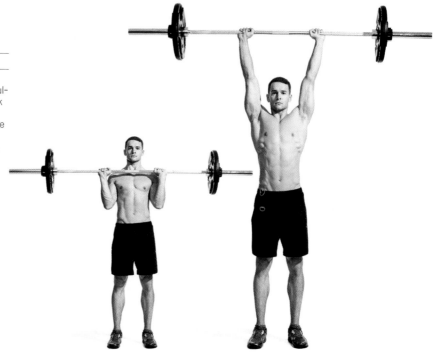

2B WEIGHTED PULLUP

SETS: 5 REPS: 5 REST: 90 SEC.

Attach a weighted belt to your waist, hold a dumbbell between your feet, or if you can't complete your reps with weight, use body weight alone. Hang from a pullup bar with hands just outside shoulder width. Pull yourself up until your chin is over the bar.

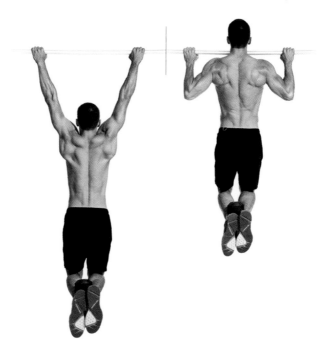

THE BEST FULL-BODY MUSCLE WORKOUT [option B]

WORKOUT #4   BY SEAN HYSON, C.S.C.S.

Applying the same principle as the previous workout, here we offer three different push, pull, and lower-body exercises with some additional ab and calf work thrown in. This routine is ideal if you find yourself with a bit more time to train than you did when choosing Option A. It can also be alternated with Option A, to add some variety to your training. The different exercise and rep ranges will switch up the muscle-building stimulus.

DIRECTIONS Alternate sets of the bench press and seated cable row. So you'll do one set of 1A, rest, then one set of 1B, rest again, and repeat until all sets are complete. Perform the remaining exercises as normal straight sets.

1A BENCH PRESS

SETS: 4 REPS: 10 REST: 60 SEC.

Grasp the bar just outside shoulder width and arch your back so there's space between your lower back and the bench. Pull the bar out of the rack and lower it to your sternum, tucking your elbows about 45 degrees to your sides. When the bar touches your body, drive your feet hard into the floor and press the bar back up.

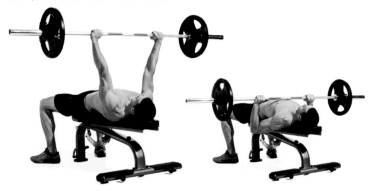

1B SEATED CABLE ROW

SETS: 4 REPS: 10 REST: 60 SEC.

Attach a straight or lat-pulldown bar to the pulley of a seated row station. Sit on the bench or floor with your feet against the foot plate and knees slightly bent. Keeping your lower back flat, bend forward at the hips to grasp the bar and row it to your sternum, squeezing your shoulder blades together in the end position. Extend your arms and feel the stretch in your back before beginning the next rep.

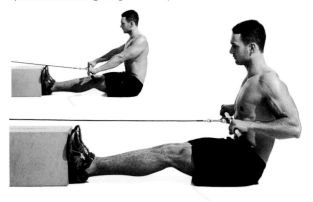

2 DUMBBELL ROMANIAN DEADLIFT

SETS: 4 REPS: 10 REST: 90 SEC.

Hold a dumbbell in each hand and stand with feet hip width. Push your hips back and, keeping your lower back in its natural arch, bend your torso forward, lowering until you feel a stretch in your hamstrings, bending slightly at the knees as needed. Squeeze your glutes as you come back up.

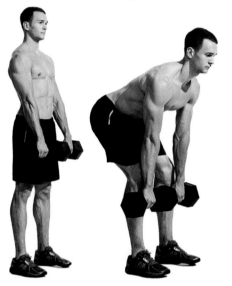

3 PALLOF PRESS ISO HOLD

SETS: 3 REPS: HOLD FOR 30 SEC. (EACH SIDE) REST: 30 SEC.

Attach a single-grip handle to a cable pulley and set it at about shoulder height. (You can also use a band.) Grasp the handle with one hand over the other and step away from the machine to put tension on the cable; turn to your left 90 degrees so your right side is now facing the machine. Stand with feet shoulder width and extend your arms in front of you. The cable will try to twist your body toward it—resist.

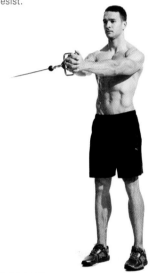

4 STANDING CALF RAISE

SETS: 4 REPS: 10 REST: 60 SEC.

Use a standing calf raise machine, or hold onto a sturdy object and stand on a block as shown. Lower your heels toward the floor until you feel a stretch in your calves. Drive the balls of your feet into the foot plate and contract your calves, raising your heels as high as possible. Control the descent on each rep.

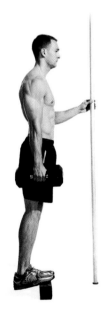
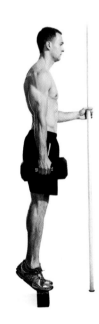

THE BEST FULL-BODY MUSCLE WORKOUT [option C]

WORKOUT #5   BY SEAN HYSON, C.S.C.S.

Here, we continue the theme of pushing, pulling, and lower-body movements making up the core of the workout and add in some direct arm work. The high-rep approach (sets of 15) works well in conjunction with the previous two sessions, and you may rotate through all three of them. For instance, perform option A on Monday, option B on Wednesday, and option C on Friday.

DIRECTIONS Perform the exercise pairs (marked "A" and "B") in alternating fashion. So you'll do one set of A, rest, then one set of B, rest again, and repeat until all sets are completed for the pair. The remaining exercises are done conventionally.

1 TRAP-BAR DEADLIFT

SETS: 3 REPS: 15 REST: 120 SEC.

Use a trap bar and stand with feet hip width. Bend your hips back and grasp the handles. Keeping your lower back in its natural arch, drive through your heels to stand up straight and extend your hips and knees.

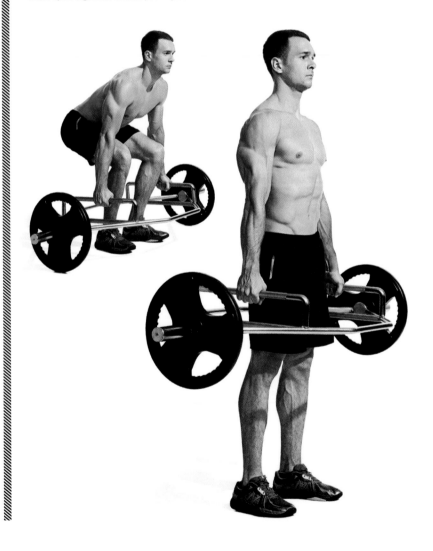

2A INCLINE DUMBBELL ROW

SETS: 3 REPS: 15 REST: 60 SEC.

Set an adjustable bench to a 30- to 45-degree incline and lie on it chest-down. Grasp a dumbbell in each hand and draw your shoulder blades back and together as you row the weights to your sides.

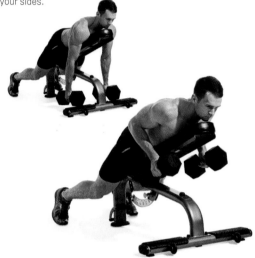

2B INCLINE DUMBBELL PRESS

SETS: 3 REPS: 15 REST: 60 SEC.

Lie back on the incline bench holding a dumbbell in each hand at shoulder level. Press the weights over your chest.

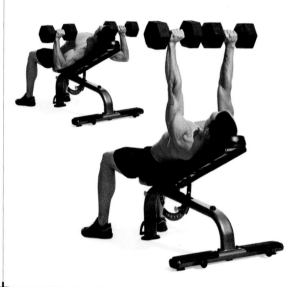

3A EZ-BAR CURL

SETS: 3 REPS: 15 REST: 60 SEC.

Grasp an EZ-curl bar at shoulder width. Keeping your upper arms stationary, curl the bar.

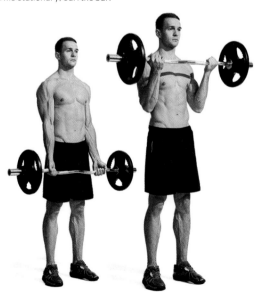

3B DECLINE EZ-BAR LYING TRICEPS EXTENSION

SETS: 3 REPS: 15 REST: 60 SEC.

Set an adjustable bench to a slight decline and lie back on it holding an EZ-curl bar at shoulder width. Press the bar over your chest and then let your upper arms drift back to about a 45-degree angle, which becomes your starting position. Bend your elbows to lower the bar behind your head, and then extend them to return to the starting position for the next rep.

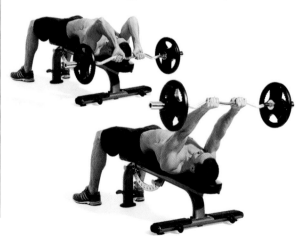

THE BEST FULL-BODY FAT-LOSS WORKOUT [option A]

WORKOUT #6   BY CRAIG RASMUSSEN, C.S.C.S.

Most big-box gyms feature a cluster of machines arranged in such a way as to provide members with a "circuit." Circuits are a gym's equivalent of a no-brainer, requiring only that the trainee move from machine to machine for a prescribed number of repetitions, over and over again.

We've got a better circuit—one that involves free weights, to build more muscle, burn more calories, and keep you challenged for the long term.

HOW IT WORKS This routine prioritizes abs by placing them first. From there, you'll move on to a light circuit that will burn loads of calories. Finally, you'll hit the main circuit, which builds strength and muscle.

DIRECTIONS Perform the first exercise as straight sets. Exercises 2A through 2D are done as a complex, so choose one pair of dumbbells and use them for each move. Use a load that allows you to complete your reps on your weakest exercise in the series. Perform six reps for each of the exercises. Rest 90 seconds and repeat.

For exercises 3A through 3D, adjust your equipment and loads as necessary, but perform them in the same circuit fashion. If you choose to repeat the workout, vary the sets and reps you perform on these last four exercises each session. This will help you to continue milking gains from the circuit for months on end. Rotate between 3 sets of 10 reps, 4 sets of 5 reps, and 2 sets of 15 reps.

1 SWISS BALL PLANK CIRCLE

SETS: 2 REPS: 30-45 SECONDS (EACH DIRECTION) REST: 60-90 SEC.

Place a Swiss ball on the floor and get into pushup position with your hands on it. Now lower your forearms to rest on the ball, keeping your entire body in a straight line with abs braced. Use your elbows to roll the ball in a circular motion, clockwise and then counter-clockwise, as if you were stirring a pot.

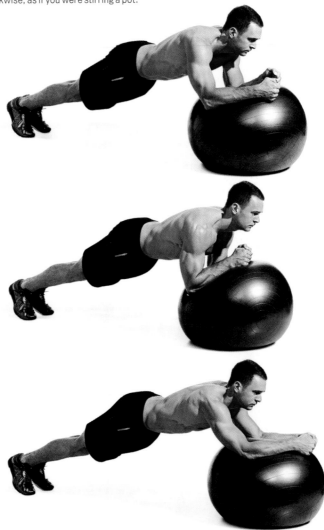

2A DUMBBELL ROMANIAN DEADLIFT

SETS: 3-5 REPS: 6 REST: 0 SEC.

Hold a dumbbell in each hand and stand with feet hip width. Push your hips back and, keeping your lower back in its natural arch, bend your torso forward. Lower your body until you feel a stretch in your hamstrings, bending slightly at the knees as needed. Squeeze your glutes as you come back up.

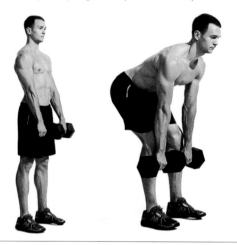

2B ALTERNATING DUMBBELL ROW

SETS: 3-5 REPS: 6 (EACH SIDE) REST: 0 SEC.

Bend forward at the hips as you did in the Romanian deadlift and row one dumbbell to your side. Lower it and repeat on the other side.

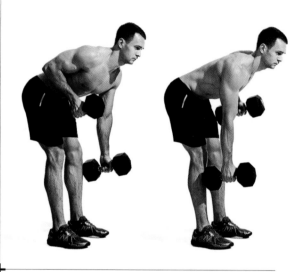

2C DUMBBELL HIGH PULL

SETS: 3-5 REPS: 6 REST: 0 SEC.

Hold dumbbells in front of your thighs and bend your knees and hips so the weights hang just above your knees. Explosively extend your hips as if jumping and pull the weights up to shoulder level with elbows wide apart, as in an upright row.

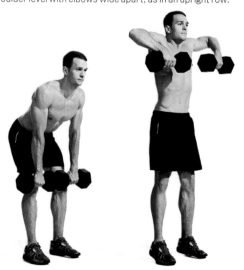

2D FRONT SQUAT TO PRESS

SETS: 3-5 REPS: 6 REST: 90 SEC.

Hold the dumbbells at shoulder level and stand with feet shoulder width. Squat as low as you can without losing the arch in your lower back. Come back up and press the weights overhead.

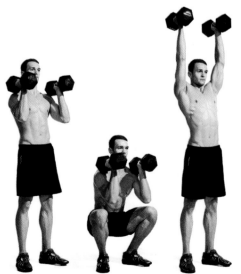

3A SNATCH-GRIP RACK DEADLIFT

SETS: 3 REPS: 10 REST: 0 SEC.

Set up as you would to deadlift, only do so in a power rack, resting the bar on the safety rods at about two inches below your knees. Grasp the bar wide, hands about double shoulder width. Extend your hips and stand up, pulling the bar to in front of your thighs.

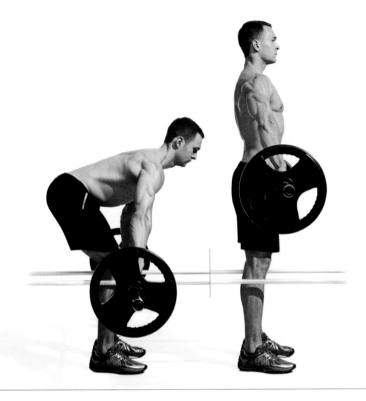

3B ALTERNATING DUMBBELL BENCH PRESS

SETS: 3 REPS: 10 (EACH SIDE) REST: 0 SEC.

Lie back on a flat bench holding dumbbells. Press them both over your chest and then lower one of them to your side. Press it up and then lower the other hand. That's one rep.

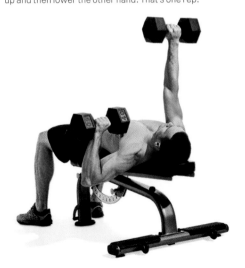

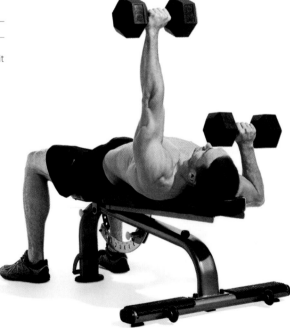

3C DUMBBELL LUNGE

SETS: 3 REPS: 10 (EACH SIDE)
REST: 0 SEC.

Stand with your feet hip width, holding a dumbbell in each hand. Step forward with one leg and lower your body until your rear knee nearly touches the floor and your front thigh is parallel to the floor.

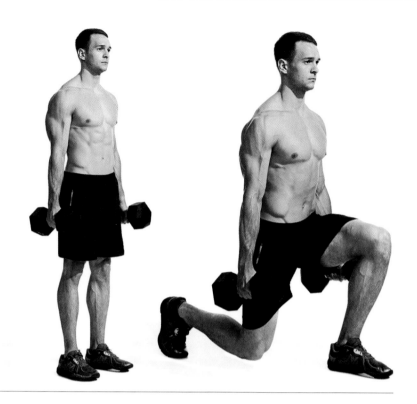

3D INVERTED ROW

SETS: 3 REPS: 10 REST: 90 SEC.

Set a barbell in a power rack (or use a Smith machine) at about hip height. Lie underneath it and grab it with hands about shoulder-width apart. Hang from the bar so your body forms a straight line. Squeeze your shoulder blades together and pull yourself up until your back is fully contracted.

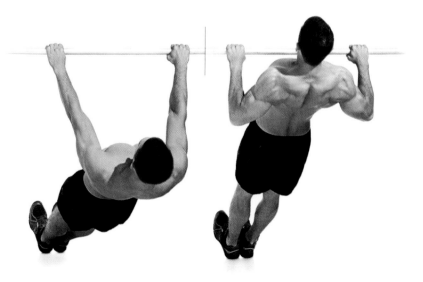

THE BEST FULL-BODY FAT LOSS WORKOUT [option B]

WORKOUT #7   BY CRAIG RASMUSSEN, C.S.C.S.

Here is another circuit that is done in the same fashion as Option A.

HOW IT WORKS Just like with Option A, this one prioritizes abs and employs a range of compound exercises to recruit more muscle groups efficiently while burning calories at a fast rate.

DIRECTIONS This routine can be substituted for Option A, or combined with it, alternating the two for a total of three sessions each week, resting a day between workouts (and then two days before repeating the cycle). Rotate the sets and reps on exercises 3A through 3D as follows: 4 sets of 5 reps, 2 sets of 15 reps, and 3 sets of 10 reps.

1 HORIZONTAL CABLE WOODCHOP

SETS: 2 REPS: 10 (EACH SIDE) REST: 60-90 SEC.

Set an adjustable cable pulley to shoulder level (or attach a band to a sturdy object) and grasp the handle with both hands. Stand with feet shoulder width apart, perpendicular to the anchor point, and arms extended, far enough away from the machine so there's tension on the cable. Twist away from the machine as if you were chopping into a tree. Keep your feet stationary.

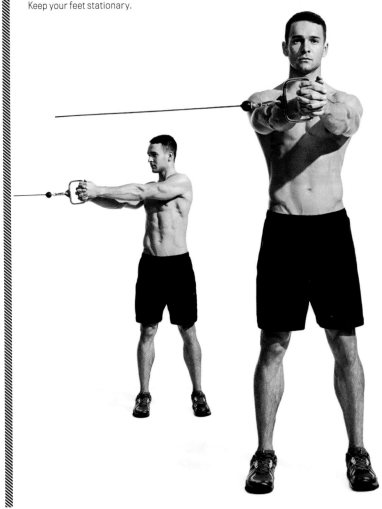

2A DEADLIFT

SETS: 3-5 REPS: 6 REST: 0 SEC.

Stand with feet about hip-width apart. Bend your hips back to reach down and grasp the bar so your hands are just outside your knees. Keeping your lower back in its natural arch, drive your heels into the floor and pull the bar up along your shins until you're standing with hips fully extended and the bar is in front of your thighs.

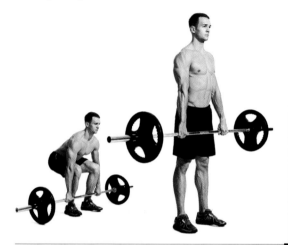

2B BENTOVER ROW

SETS: 3-5 REPS: 6 REST: 0 SEC.

Grasp the bar overhand at shoulder width and let it hang in front of your thighs. Bend at the hips and lower your torso until it's nearly parallel to the floor. Bend your knees a bit to take tension off your hamstrings. Squeeze your shoulder blades together and pull the bar to your belly.

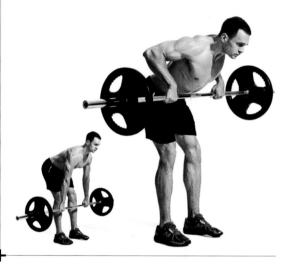

2C HANG CLEAN

SETS: 3-5 REPS: 6 REST: 0 SEC.

Hold the bar at shoulder width in front of your thighs and bend your hips and knees so that the bar lowers to just above your knees. Now explosively extend your hips as if jumping while at the same time shrugging your shoulders and pulling the bar straight up in front of your torso. As the bar reaches chest level, bend your elbows so that your palms face the ceiling and catch the bar at shoulder level, upper arms parallel to the floor. Bend your hips and knees as you catch the bar to absorb the impact and then stand up straight.

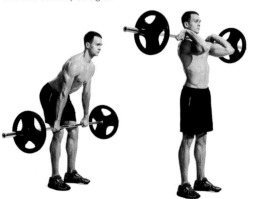

2D PUSH PRESS

SETS: 3-5 REPS: 6 REST: 90 SEC.

Hold the bar at shoulder level. Dip your knees to gather momentum and then extend them explosively to press the weight overhead.

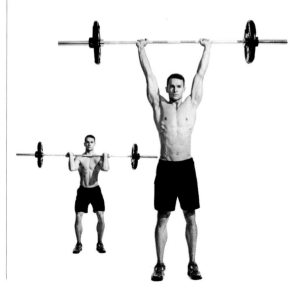

3A SQUAT

SETS: 4 REPS: 5 REST: 0 SEC.

Set up in a squat rack or cage. Grasp the bar as far apart as is comfortable and step under it. Squeeze your shoulder blades together and nudge the bar out of the rack. Step back and stand with your feet shoulder width and your toes turned slightly outward. Take a deep breath and bend your hips back and then bend your knees to lower your body as far as you can without losing the arch in your lower back. Push your knees outward as you descend. Extend your hips to come back up, continuing to push your knees outward.

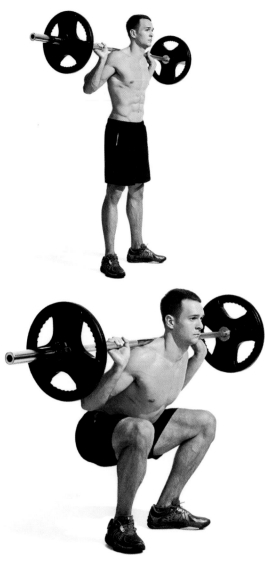

3B OVERHEAD PRESS

SETS: 4 REPS: 5 REST: 0 SEC.

Perform as you did the push press but keep your knees straight and press the bar overhead strictly. Keep your abs braced and squeeze the bar tight throughout.

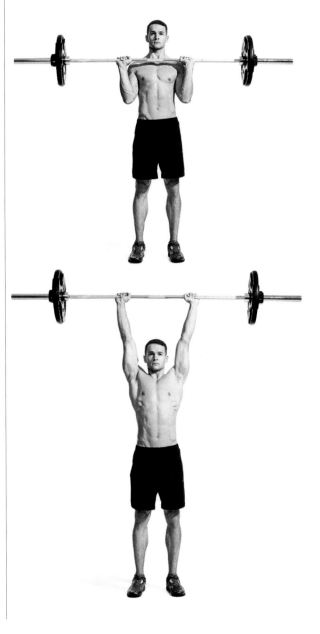

3C SINGLE-LEG ROMANIAN DEADLIFT

SETS: 4 REPS: 5 (EACH SIDE) REST: 0 SEC.

Hold a dumbbell in one hand and stand on the opposite leg. Bend your hips back and lower your torso until you feel your lower back is about to lose its arch. Squeeze your glutes and extend your hips to come up.

3D CHINUP

SETS: 4 REPS: 5 REST: 90 SEC.

Grasp a chinup bar underhand at shoulder width. Hang from the bar and then pull yourself up until your chin is over it.

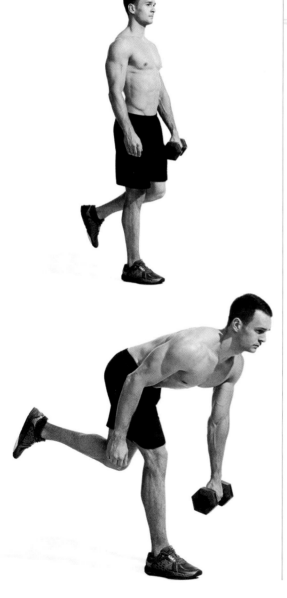

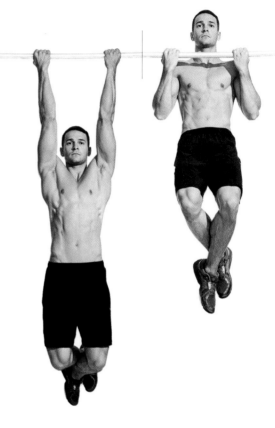

04 BARBELL

Because of its association with bench pressing, squatting, and deadlifting, the barbell tends to be thought of as a tool that's good only for performing specific lifts or hitting one muscle group at a time. In later chapters we'll show you how to get great workouts for any body part with a barbell alone, but here we've got routines that work your whole body.

You don't necessarily need a bench, a rack, or even two matched plates to get a good workout with a barbell. A corner of a room in which you can wedge one end can be enough. And if you use the Olympic lifts—the exercises contested in Olympic weightlifting competitions—you can hit every major muscle of the body in minutes. These are just two of the approaches you're about to discover.

THE BEST BARBELL-ONLY WORKOUT [option A]

WORKOUT #8   BY JOE STANKOWSKI, C.P.T.

If you train at home or anywhere else that provides only a barbell and a small amount of weight, you can make the most of it by speeding or slowing your reps and performing your exercises circuit-style.

HOW IT WORKS The barbell was invented to carry balanced loads but works just as well out of balance. The following exercises can be performed with one end wedged between two walls while you lift the other end like a lever. You may find that pressing the bar like a lever feels less stressful to your shoulders, plus it activates your core to a greater degree.

DIRECTIONS Perform the exercises as a circuit, completing one set of each in turn without rest. If an exercise feels easy using the load you have available, perform your reps slower and with more control. (Or, if you have extra weight, load it.) Another option is to choke down on the bar. Gripping it lower will decrease your mechanical advantage and make the exercise harder.
  After the last exercise, rest two minutes and then repeat the entire circuit. Continue for 20 minutes. You can repeat the workout up to four times per week, resting a day between sessions.

1 SPLIT SQUAT TO PRESS

REPS: 10-12 (EACH SIDE) REST: 0 SEC.

Wedge the end of the barbell into a corner of the room (to avoid damage to the walls, you may have to wrap a towel around it). Load the opposite end with a weight plate and grasp it toward the end. Get into a lunge position with your left leg in front, bent to where your thigh is parallel to the floor and your right knee nearly touches the floor. Stand up explosively and press the bar straight up.

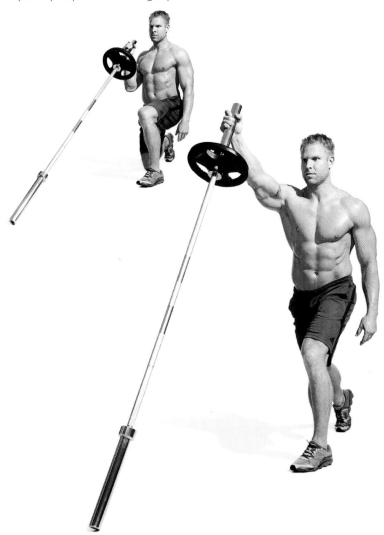

2 SINGLE-ARM ROW W/ PARTIAL LUNGE

REPS: 10-12 (EACH SIDE) REST: 0 SEC.

Hold the barbell behind the sleeve (where you load the weights) with your left hand. Get into a lunge position but not deep—keep both legs slightly extended so that the bar and plate don't brush the floor. Draw your shoulder blade back and row the bar to your ribs.

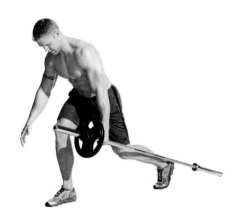
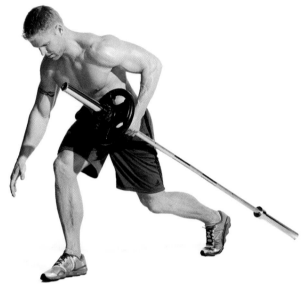

3 BARBELL RUSSIAN TWIST

REPS: 10-12 (EACH SIDE) REST: 0 SEC.

Grasp the bar near the very end again—this time with both hands. Stand with feet shoulder width. Swing the bar to your left, pivoting your feet as needed, and then swing to your right.

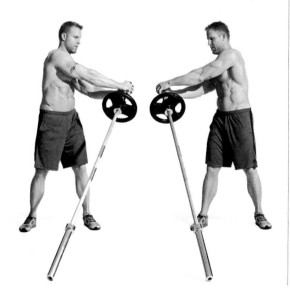

4 LEVER FLOOR PRESS

REPS: 10-12 (EACH SIDE) REST: 120 SEC.

Lie on your back on the floor and grasp the end of the bar again behind the sleeve with your left hand. Hold it just above your shoulder and extend your right arm out to your side for support. Press the bar over your chest.

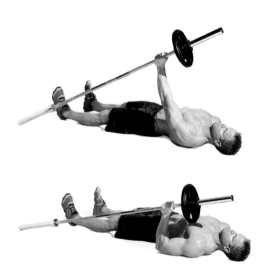

THE BEST BARBELL-ONLY WORKOUT [option B]

WORKOUT #9   BY BRIAN GRASSO

Call this one the "No Excuses Workout" because we have yet to hear a compelling reason why someone can't succeed with it. First of all, it takes only six minutes to complete. Second, it requires just a barbell and a pair of plates. Load the bar once and you're ready to go. Think you can handle that?

HOW IT WORKS The workout is a barbell complex—a series of exercises that flow. The finish position of the hang clean sets you up perfectly for the front squat, which then allows you to move right into the overhead press, and so on.

Choose one weight, which will be determined by the exercise you can lift the least amount on (in this case, the overhead lunge), and go for it. The pace will be so intense that you'll be grateful the workout is over in six minutes. Fortunately, your metabolism will remain accelerated for 48 hours afterward.

DIRECTIONS Perform the exercises as a circuit, completing one set of each in turn without rest. Complete three reps for each move. Time your circuit. After the last exercise, check your timer and rest as long as it took you to perform the circuit. Repeat for three total circuits.

Choose a load you could use for 10 reps on a normal overhead press, and keep that same weight for all the exercises.

1 ROMANIAN DEADLIFT

REPS: 3 REST: 0 SEC.

Hold the bar at shoulder width and stand with feet hip width. Bend your hips back as far as you can. Allow your knees to bend as needed while you lower the bar along your shins until you feel a stretch in your hamstrings. Keep your lower back arched throughout. Squeeze your glutes as you come back up.

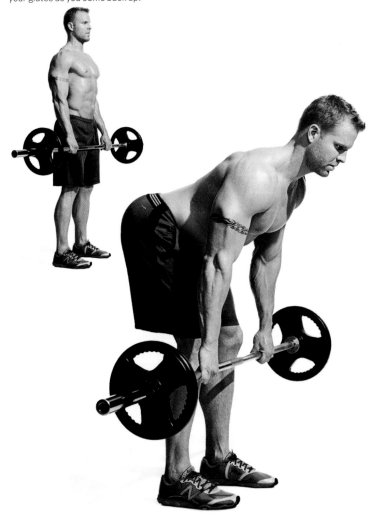

2 HANG CLEAN

REPS: 3 REST: 0 SEC.

With the bar in front of your thighs, bend your hips and knees so that the bar lowers to just above your knees. Now explosively extend your hips as if jumping while at the same time shrugging your shoulders and pulling the bar straight up in front of your torso. As the bar reaches chest level, bend your elbows so that your palms face the ceiling and catch the bar at shoulder level. Bend your hips and knees as you catch the bar to absorb the impact.

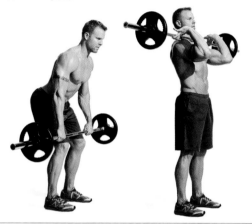

3 FRONT SQUAT

REPS: 3 REST: 0 SEC.

From the catch position of the hang clean, squat as low as you can without losing the arch in your lower back.

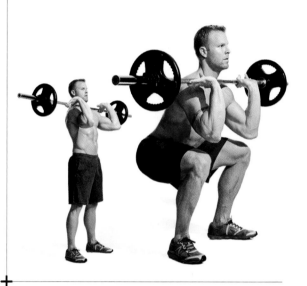

4 OVERHEAD PRESS

REPS: 3 REST: 0 SEC.

From standing, press the bar overhead, pushing your head forward and shrugging your traps as the bar passes your face.

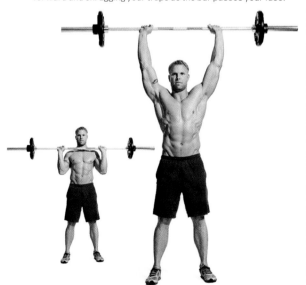

5 OVERHEAD LUNGE

REPS: 3 (EACH SIDE) REST: SEE DIRECTIONS

Hold the bar overhead and step forward with your left leg. Lower yourself until your left thigh is parallel to the floor and your rear knee nearly touches the floor.

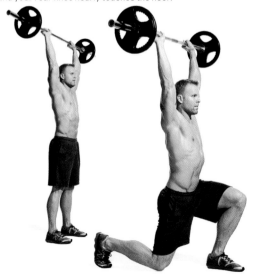

05 DUMBBELLS & KETTLEBELLS

Ever since the reemergence of the kettlebell as a training staple about a decade ago, there's been a debate over which is superior, dumbbells or kettlebells. While this argument is pretty much a stalemate, we'll take kettlebells.

For one, kettlebells have thicker handles, so your grip and forearms are recruited more heavily. For another, the bell hangs at a distance from the handle, so the load is offset, which makes every move more difficult to stabilize and more demanding of your core to provide that stability. Furthermore, just about any exercise you can think to do with a dumbbell can be replicated with a kettlebell and will feel much harder.

But, hey, people have been getting ripped sans kettlebells for years, so if dumbbells are all you have, forget what you read above. Dumbbells tend to take up less space and are a little more convenient to store, and they're certainly more common and easy to find, so you might as well learn how to make the most of them.

This chapter explores your options when training conditions are most dire—when you have access only to embarrassingly light weights, mismatched weights, or even just one weight. All the workouts that follow can be performed with either dumbbells or kettlebells. Or, a single bell, as the case may be.

THE BEST TWO-DUMBBELL/ KETTLEBELL WORKOUT [option A]

WORKOUT #10   BY JOE STANKOWSKI, C.P.T.

Whether you're visiting relatives or in a hotel with an underwhelming "fitness center," there may come a time when all you have access to is a measly pair of dumbbells or kettlebells. Not a problem, now that you have this routine.

HOW IT WORKS In this situation, the load you have will be more appropriate for some exercises than others. To see that you get the most out of the workout we prescribe here, whatever the poundage you have to work with, you'll need to adjust the speed of your reps. A pair of 25-pound dumbbells, for example, probably won't be challenging on exercises such as the stepup. In this case, perform your reps more slowly to test your endurance and build muscle control. On other exercises, like the bentover lateral raise, 25 pounds may be just right or a bit heavy, so perform your reps explosively.

If you should happen to have two unevenly weighted dumbbells, such as a 25-pounder and a 15-pounder, don't be discouraged. Simply switch the weights in your hands each time you repeat the circuit. Asymmetrical loads force your core to stabilize you even more on each exercise.

DIRECTIONS Perform the exercises as a circuit, completing one set of each in turn without rest. After the last exercise, rest two minutes and then repeat. Continue for 20 minutes. You can repeat the workout up to four times per week.

1 SIDE PLANK W/ LATERAL RAISE

SETS: AS MANY AS POSSIBLE REPS: 10-12 (EACH SIDE) REST: 0 SEC.

Lie on your left side resting your left forearm on the floor for support. Hold the dumbbell in your right hand. Raise your hips up so that your body forms a straight line and brace your abs—your weight should be on your left forearm and the edge of your left foot. From this position, raise the weight in your right hand until your arm is parallel to the floor. If the dumbbell or kettlebell you have is too heavy to perform a lateral raise with in this position, you can use a weight plate from the dumbbell (if it's the plate-loaded kind), or simply skip the lateral raise and use the weight to resist your side plank.

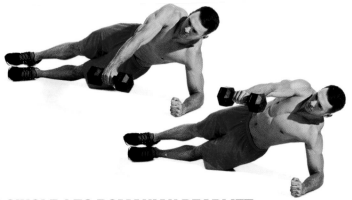

2 SINGLE-LEG ROMANIAN DEADLIFT

SETS: AS MANY AS POSSIBLE REPS: 10-12 (EACH SIDE) REST: 0 SEC.

Hold a dumbbell in one hand and stand on the opposite leg. Bend your hips back and lower your torso until you feel your lower back is about to lose its arch. Squeeze your glutes and extend your hips to come up.

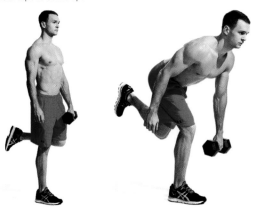

3 DUMBBELL PUSHUP W/ ROW

SETS: AS MANY AS POSSIBLE REPS: 10–12 (EACH SIDE)
REST: 0 SEC.

Get into pushup position with a dumbbell in each hand. Perform a pushup and then, in the up position, shift your weight to your right side and row the left-hand dumbbell to your side. Perform another pushup, shift your weight to the left, and row with the right hand.

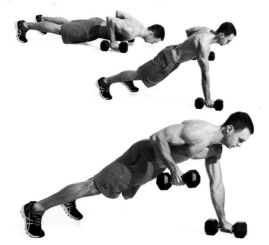

4 STEPUP

SETS: AS MANY AS POSSIBLE REPS: 10–12 (EACH SIDE)
REST: 0 SEC.

Stand behind a bench or other elevated surface that will put your thigh at parallel to the floor when you place your foot onto it. Hold a dumbbell in each hand and step up onto the bench but leave your trailing leg hanging off.

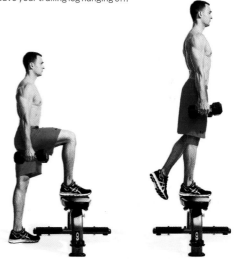

5 BENTOVER LATERAL RAISE

SETS: AS MANY AS POSSIBLE REPS: 10–12 REST: 0 SEC.

Hold the dumbbells and stand with feet shoulder width. Bend your hips back and, keeping your lower back in its natural arch, lower your torso until it's parallel to the floor. Allow your arms to hang. Squeeze your shoulder blades together and raise your arms out to the sides until they're parallel to the floor.

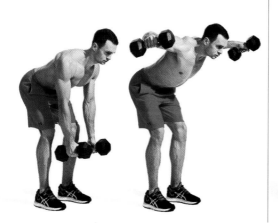

6 LUNGE W/ OVERHEAD PRESS

SETS: AS MANY AS POSSIBLE REPS: 10–12 (EACH SIDE)
REST: 120 SEC.

Hold the dumbbells at shoulder level and step forward into a lunge, lowering your body until your rear knee nearly touches the floor and your front thigh is parallel to the floor. Push off your front foot to come back to the starting position and then press the weights overhead.

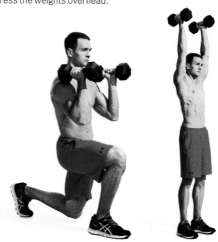

THE BEST TWO-DUMBBELL/ KETTLEBELL WORKOUT [option B]

WORKOUT #11   BY SEAN HYSON, C.S.C.S.

A hotel or home gym outfitted with just a small dumbbell rack can easily become a torture chamber with a little creativity. High reps, circuits, and supersets (two exercises done back to back with no rest) can make even the lightest weights feel heavy after a while and make the workout double as a cardio session.

HOW IT WORKS The biggest obstacle you're likely to face with nothing but dumbbells at your disposal is a lack of weight to make your legs work hard. This workout's fast pace will help to offset that, and so will working one leg at a time. Be prepared to switch to lighter dumbbells on subsequent circuits when the fatigue really kicks in. If you have only one pair of dumbbells, ignore the rep ranges on everything but the Bulgarian split squat and stepup, and go for as many reps as possible each set.

DIRECTIONS Perform exercises 1A through 1C as a circuit. So, you'll do one set of the Bulgarian split squat, one set of stepups, and then one set of the dumbbell squat before resting for two minutes. Repeat until all the prescribed sets are complete. Perform the remaining paired exercises (2A and 2B, 3A and 3B) as supersets. That means you'll do a set of A and then a set of B before resting, and repeat until all sets are completed for the pair. The last exercise, the pushup, is done as conventional straight sets.

1A BULGARIAN SPLIT SQUAT

SETS: 2-3 REPS: 15-20 (EACH SIDE) REST: 0 SEC.

Stand lunge-length in front of a bench. Hold a dumbbell in each hand and rest the top of your left foot on the bench behind you. Lower your body until your rear knee nearly touches the floor and your front thigh is parallel to the floor.

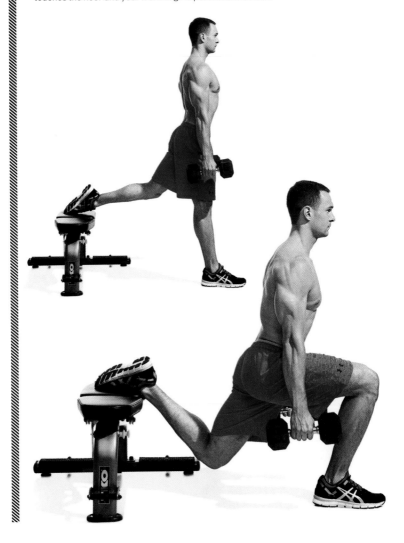

1B STEPUP

SETS: 2-3 REPS: 15-20 (EACH SIDE) REST: 0 SEC.

Stand behind a bench or other elevated surface that will put your thigh at parallel to the floor when you place your foot onto it. Hold a dumbbell in each hand and step up onto the bench but leave your trailing leg hanging off.

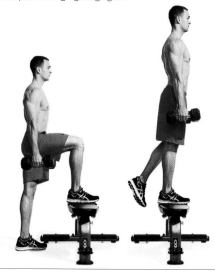

1C DUMBBELL SQUAT

SETS: 2-3 REPS: AS MANY AS POSSIBLE REST: 120 SEC.

Hold dumbbells at shoulder level and stand with your feet shoulder width. Sit back with your hips and lower your body as far as you can without losing the arch in your lower back.

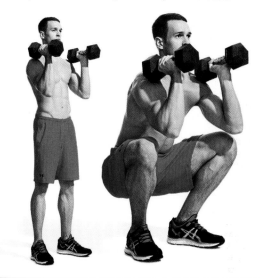

2A ELBOW-OUT DUMBBELL ROW

SETS: 2-3 REPS: 15-20 REST: 0 SEC.

Keeping your lower back arched, bend your hips back until your torso is parallel to the floor. Turn your palms to face your legs, squeeze your shoulder blades together, and row the dumbbells—raising your arms out 90 degrees from your torso.

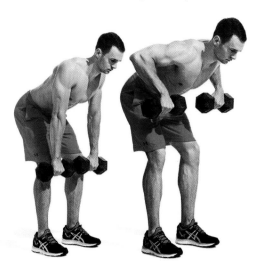

2B DUMBBELL OVERHEAD PRESS

SETS: 2-3 REPS: 15-20
REST: 90 SEC.

Hold a dumbbell in each hand at shoulder level with palms facing in front of you. Brace your abs and press the weights overhead.

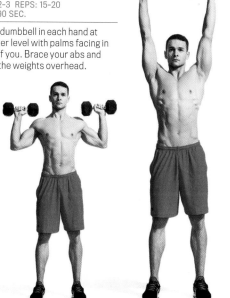

3A ONE-ARM, ELBOW-IN DUMBBELL ROW

SETS: 2-3 REPS: 15-20 (EACH SIDE) REST: 0 SEC.

Perform a row as directed previously, but use one arm at a time and draw your elbow straight back so you row the weight to your side with palm facing in.

3B ONE-ARM, ELBOW-IN DUMBBELL OVERHEAD PRESS

SETS: 2-3 REPS: 15-20 (EACH SIDE) REST: 90 SEC.

Perform an overhead press as directed previously, but use one arm at a time and turn your palm to face in.

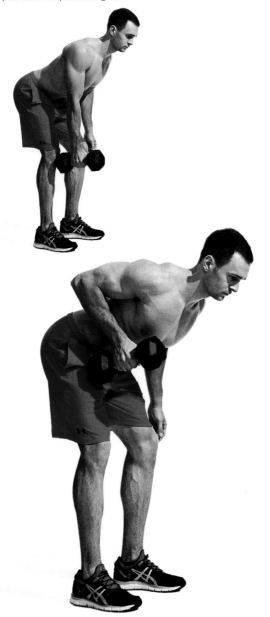

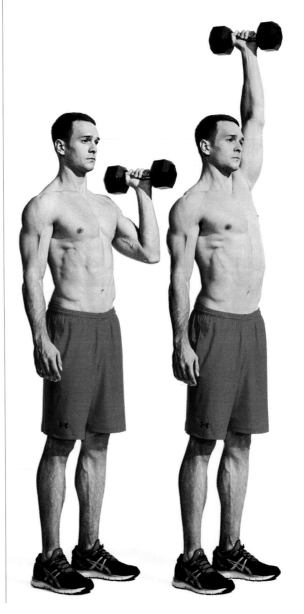

4 PUSHUP

SETS: 2-3 REPS: AS MANY AS POSSIBLE REST: 60 SEC.

Place your hands on the floor at shoulder width. Keeping your abs braced and your body in a straight line, squeeze your shoulder blades together and lower your body until your chest is an inch above the floor.

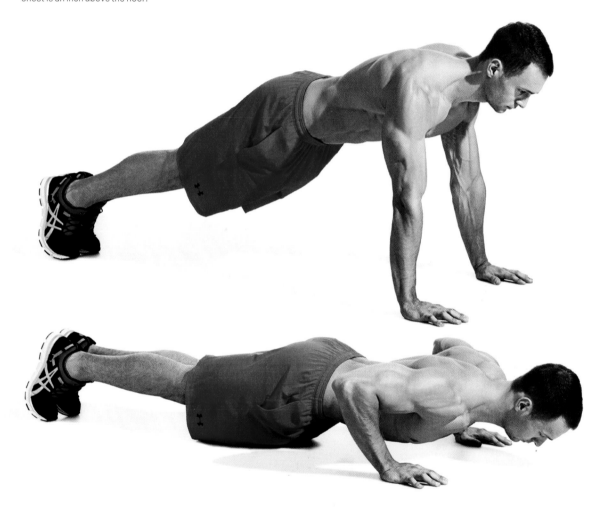

THE BEST ONE-DUMBBELL/ KETTLEBELL WORKOUT

WORKOUT #12   BY C.J. MURPHY, M.F.S.

As trendy as kettlebells have become, many chain gyms don't offer enough that you can be sure you'll get a matching pair at a given time (especially if that time is during peak hours). Your best bet then is to do what you can with a single kettlebell.

Incidentally, if you train at home and have just one dumbbell that you've been using as a paperweight up until now, this workout applies equally to you (kettlebells and dumbbells can be used interchangeably).

HOW IT WORKS One bell offers a distinct set of benefits from a pair. Your body will have to compensate for the imbalance by recruiting your core muscles more intensely, and working one side at a time will make for longer sets with a greater cardiovascular demand. Done as a circuit, the exercises that follow raise your heart rate even further, making this workout a great adjunct to a strict diet for fat loss.

DIRECTIONS The workout consists of two circuits. In Circuit 1, you'll perform the exercises in sequence for six reps each. Complete as many rounds as possible in six minutes, and then rest one minute. Repeat twice more and then rest two minutes before beginning Circuit 2.

▼ CIRCUIT 1

1 ONE-ARM SNATCH

REPS: 6 (EACH SIDE) REST: 0 SEC.

Hold a kettlebell in front of your thighs with your right hand and stand with feet between hip and shoulder width. Keep your torso as upright as possible and bend your knees until the weight hangs at mid-shin level—maintain the arch in your lower back. Jump, extending your hips explosively, and raise the weight straight up your body. When it gets to your chest, flip your wrist and "catch" the bell overhead with arm extended.

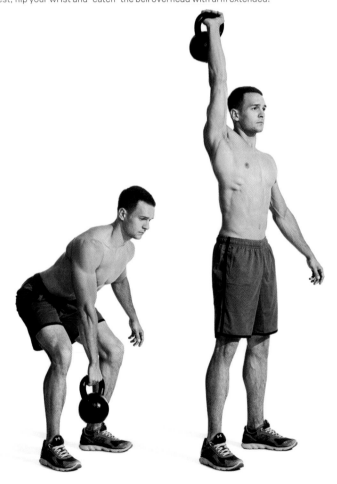

2 KETTLEBELL PRESS-OUT

REPS: 6 REST: 0 SEC.

Hold the weight close to your chest at shoulder level with both hands on the handle and palms facing each other. Squat down as deeply as you can and then press the bell straight out in front of you with arms extended. Bring it back to your chest and repeat for reps while maintaining the squat position.

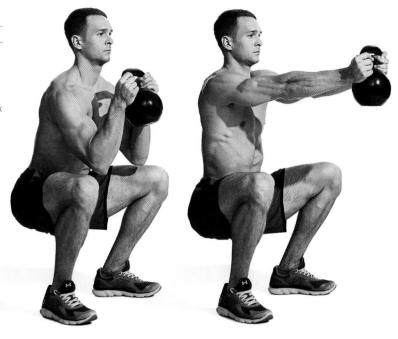

3 HARD-STYLE KETTLEBELL SWING

REPS: 6 REST: 0 SEC.

Stand with feet hip-width apart and the weight on the floor. Grasp the kettlebell with both hands (palms facing you) and, keeping your lower back flat, extend your hips to raise it off the floor. From there, take a deep breath and bend your hips back, allowing the weight to swing back between your legs. Explosively extend your hips and exhale—allowing the momentum to swing the weight up to shoulder level. Control the descent, but use the momentum to begin the next rep.

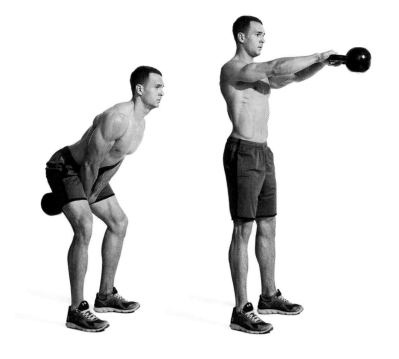

▼ CIRCUIT 2

TURKISH GETUP

Lie on your back on the floor holding a kettlebell with your right hand over your chest, arm perpendicular to the floor. Bend your right knee 90 degrees and plant your foot on the floor. Brace your abs and raise your torso off the floor. Use your left hand for support. Now use your right foot to raise your hips off the floor. Sweep your left leg back and rest on your left knee. Come up to a standing position, and then reverse the motion to return to the floor. Note that the foot that rests on the floor changes with the hand that's holding the weight (when you perform the getup with the left hand, your left foot will lie flat).

Perform one rep with the weight in your right hand and then immediately switch hands and repeat. Switch back to your right hand and do two reps. Then do two on your left. Continue adding one extra rep in this fashion until you're up to five on each side. Without rest, reverse the process and work back down to one rep.

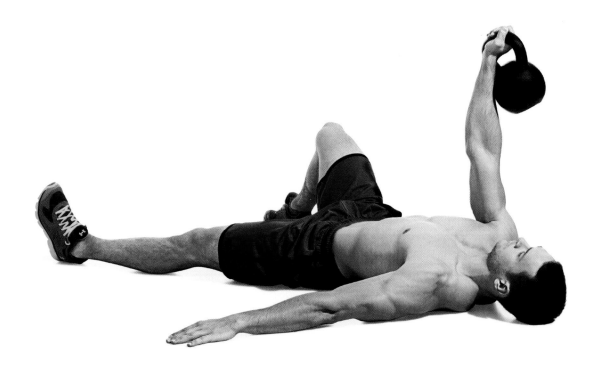

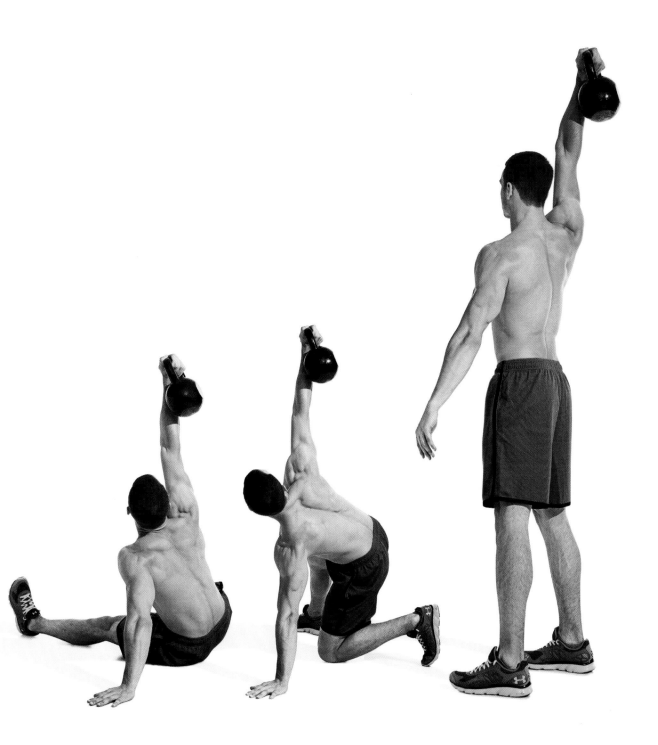

06 MACHINES

We've never been big fans of machines at *Men's Fitness*. For most people, they represent taking the path of least resistance—literally. Machines determine your range of motion and the way your muscles move the weight, so you don't train your body to do these things. If you're just getting into lifting and want to gain weight and get stronger, machines aren't the best way to go. But if you're older and have nagging injuries, or you want to isolate one muscle at a time to bring it up, machines may be your best weapons.

Of course, you may find yourself in a situation where it's machines or bust, as in the case of some hotel gyms and community fitness centers. In any event, you can get just as hard a workout with machinery as you can with iron.

A note here: Whenever possible, we'd prefer you do your machine exercises on Hammer Strength equipment (*life fitness.com*). This is a quality brand that offers a unique feature—isolateral movement. That means you can lift each limb independently. In this way, Hammer Strength equipment follows your unique biomechanics, letting your limbs work in their natural fashion, rather than having to conform to the narrower paths that most machines set.

THE BEST ALL-MACHINE WORKOUT

WORKOUT #13   BY JASON FERRUGGIA

There are three likely reasons you would do a workout entirely with machines. One is that you fear free weights. Another is that you're in a hotel gym with machines as your only workout options, and the third is that you're a little beat up and need to protect overworked joints or work around nagging injuries. Whatever the case may be, machines are suitable muscle-building equipment, and you can train your whole body with them.

HOW IT WORKS This workout uses a classic bodybuilding approach: pyramid sets. You start with higher reps and increase the weight slightly each set while reducing reps to gradually warm up the muscles and joints and recruit more and more muscle fibers. No matter how hard you train or how heavy you go, you're unlikely to get injured, because the machines are stabilizing the load for you. This isn't always ideal, but it does allow you to push yourself and focus your mind solely on the muscles you want to work without worrying about a freak accident keeping you out of the gym for weeks.

DIRECTIONS Perform the exercise pairs (marked "A" and "B") as alternating sets. So you'll do a set of A, rest, then a set of B, rest again, and continue for all the prescribed sets. The remaining exercises are done as conventional straight sets.

1A CHEST PRESS

SETS: 3 REPS: 12, 10, 8 REST: 60 SEC.

Adjust the height of the seat so that the handles are in line with the middle of your chest. When you grasp the handles, your elbows should be bent nearly 90 degrees. Press the handles until your elbows are locked out. Keep tension on your muscles at the bottom of each rep.

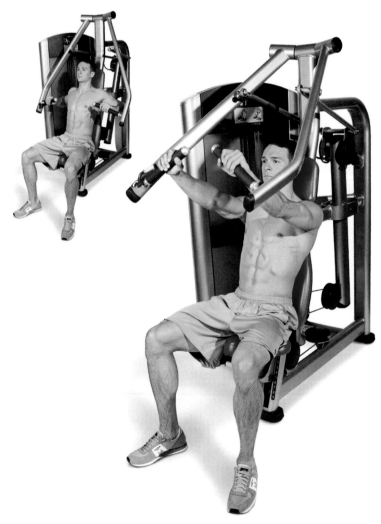

1B CHEST-SUPPORTED ROW

SETS: 3 REPS: 12, 10, 8 REST: 60 SEC.

Using a chest-supported row machine, row the weight to your belly, squeezing your shoulder blades together at the top of the movement.

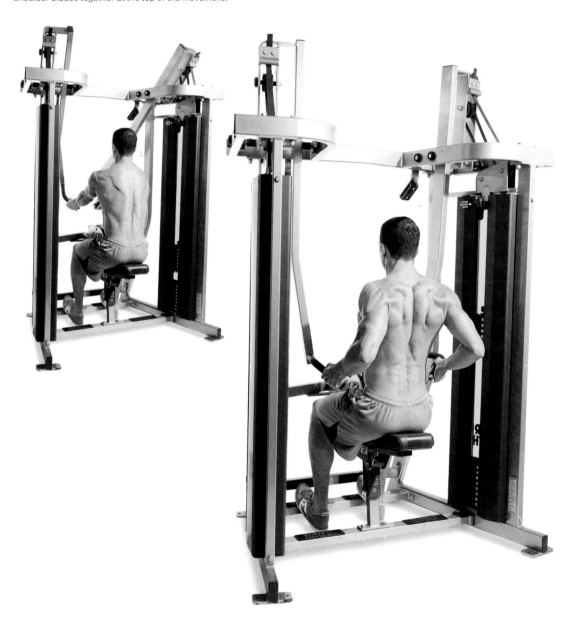

2A SHOULDER PRESS

SETS: 3 REPS: 12, 10, 8 REST: 60 SEC.

Adjust the seat of a shoulder press machine so that the handles are at shoulder level. If you have shoulder problems, and if your machine allows it, grasp the handles so your palms face each other. Otherwise, grasp them with palms facing forward as normal. Make sure your elbows track in a normal pressing path as you press the handles overhead.

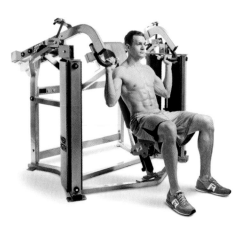
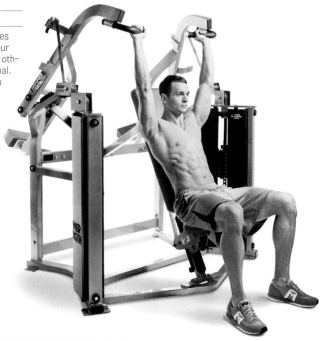

2B NEUTRAL-GRIP PULLDOWN

SETS: 3 REPS: 15, 12, 10 REST: 60 SEC.

Attach a close-grip V-handle to the pulley of a lat-pulldown machine, or use two single-grip handles as shown. Grasp the handle so your palms face each other and set your legs under the pad. Pull the handle to your collarbone, driving your elbows down and back.

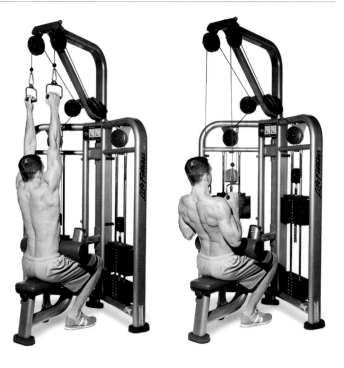

3 CALF RAISE ON LEG PRESS

SETS: 3 REPS: 25, 20, 15   REST: 60 SEC.

Set up in a leg press machine and place your feet at the bottom of
the foot plate at shoulder width so that only the balls of your feet
are on the plate. Remove the safeties and allow the weight to flex
your ankles slowly until you feel a stretch in your calves. Extend
your ankles to raise the weight back up.

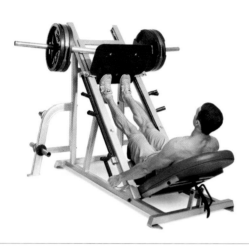
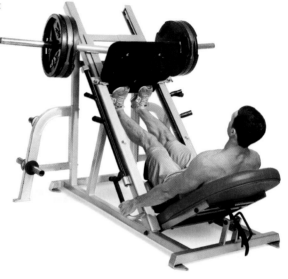

4 LEG PRESS

SETS: 4 REPS: 25, 20, 15, 10 REST: 120 SEC.

Adjust the seat of the machine so that you can sit comfortably
with your hips beneath your knees and your knees in line with
your feet. Remove the safeties and lower your knees toward
your chest until they're bent 90 degrees and then press back up.
Be careful not to go too low or you risk your lower back coming
off the seat (which can cause injury).

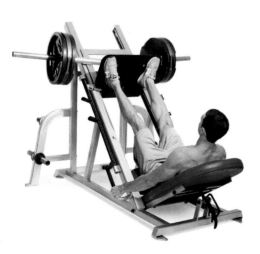
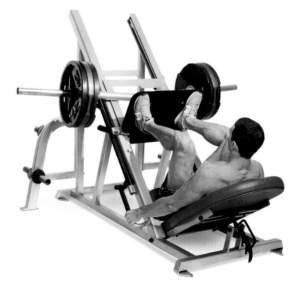

07 **BANDS**

The elastic exercise band tends to get lumped in with the Body Bar, aerobics step, and Shake Weight as so-called "wussy" equipment, while the barbell and dumbbell are beyond reproach. But this isn't a fair judgment, especially if you're using high-quality bands.

We like the loop bands that *Elitefts.net* sells. They're durable and can be used for multiple purposes and numerous exercises. If a cheap one is all you have, you can make do, but Elite's bands are a good investment, especially if you plan on traveling a lot. Lightweight and compact, they allow you to take your workouts with you.

What bands provide that no other equipment (except cables) can is accommodating resistance. Take the pushup, for example. The closer you get to locking out your elbows, the easier the exercise feels. The movement feels hardest when your chest is close to the floor. Adding resistance to the pushup with a band will intensify the last few inches of the move—as the band gets more stretched out—making you work harder, and there's nothing wussy about that.

THE BEST FULL-BODY BAND WORKOUT

WORKOUT #14   BY BEN BRUNO

This workout gets your blood moving. In fact, it makes it run up and down your body as you alternate between upper- and lower-body exercises, forcing your heart to work extra hard, which in turn, stimulates calorie burning. The result is increased strength and conditioning while trimming fat.

HOW IT WORKS The exercises are grouped into "non-competing" mini-circuits. This means that they work different areas of the body so muscle fatigue isn't carried over from one move to the next. For instance, following up a pushup with a good morning won't make your chest any more tired, so you can give each exercise your full effort and strength. Your heart, however, experiences the opposite effect. With blood racing back and forth to different muscles, your heart rate is constantly elevated. This leads to more calories burned during the workout and greater fat loss afterward.

DIRECTIONS Perform the exercise groups in sequence. So you'll do one set of A, B, and C, resting as prescribed between them, and then repeat until all the prescribed sets for that group are completed. Note that the last group is just two exercises, though done in the same fashion. Make sure you have a few different band options so you can use the appropriate tension on each exercise.

1A PUSHUP

SETS: 4 REPS: 10-12 REST: 60 SEC.

Grasp the end of a band in one hand and wrap it around your back. Get into pushup position with your hands shoulder width and your core braced. Pin both hands to the floor with the ends of the band in your palms and perform pushups.

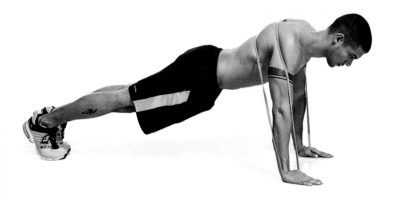
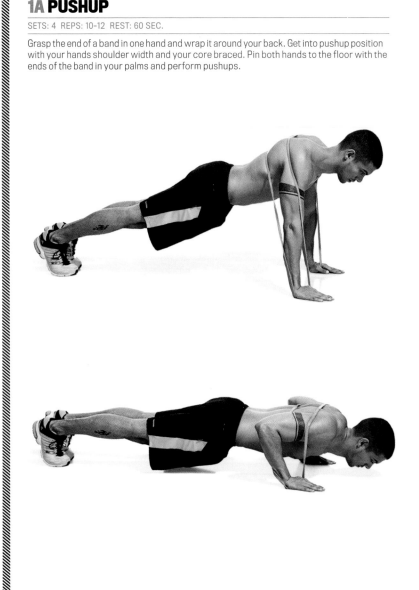

1B GOOD MORNING

SETS: 4 REPS: 12 REST: 60 SEC.

Stand on the band and loop the other end over the back of your neck and stand tall. Keeping your lower back in its natural arch, bend your hips back and lower your torso until it's nearly parallel to the floor. Think about keeping your chest up and pointing forward. Explosively extend your hips to come back up.

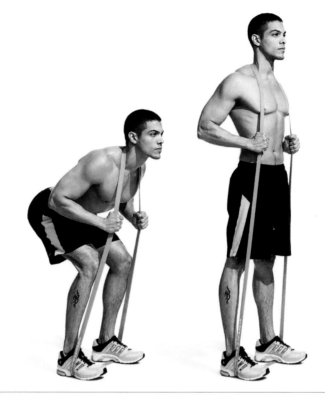

1C PULL APART

SETS: 4 REPS: 10 REST: 60 SEC.

Stand on and grasp a band loop, or a single tube as shown, hands shoulder width. Keeping your arms straight, raise your arms in front of your body to shoulder level. Now, without letting your arms drop, draw your arms out 90 degrees to your sides as if you were pulling the tube apart. Squeeze your shoulder blades together.

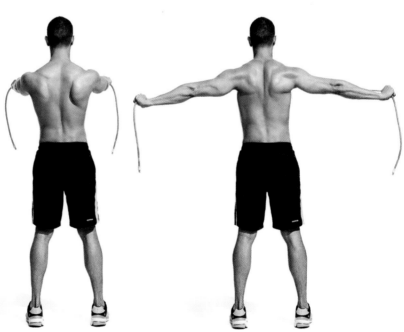

2A SQUAT

SETS: 4 REPS: 20 REST: 60 SEC.

Stand on the band or tube with feet shoulder width and toes turned slightly out. Grasp the ends of the band in each hand and hold them at shoulder level with palms facing you. Bend your hips back and squat down as low as you can without losing the arch in your lower back. Explosively extend your hips to come back up.

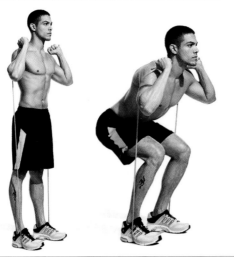

2B BAND ROW

SETS: 4 REPS: 15 REST: 60 SEC.

Attach the band to a doorknob or other sturdy object of similar height. Hold the opposite end in both hands and stand back from the door so you feel tension on the band. Row the band to your belly.

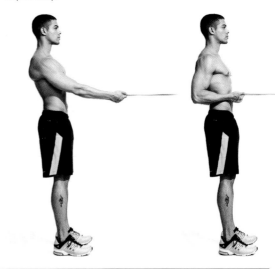

2C PALLOF PRESS

SETS: 4 REPS: 10 (EACH SIDE)
REST: 60 SEC.

Attach the band to a sturdy object at stomach level. Hold the other end with both hands and step away from the attachment point, turning your body perpendicular to it to put tension on the band. Pull the band in front of your chest and then press it out with arms straight. Bend your arms and draw your hands back toward you, resisting the band from twisting your torso. That's one rep.

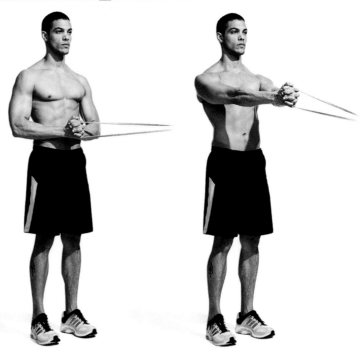

3A TRICEPS PUSHDOWN

SETS: 4 REPS: 20 REST: 60 SEC.

Attach the band to a sturdy overhead object
and grasp the free end with both hands. Tuck
your elbows to your sides and extend your
elbows to lock them out.

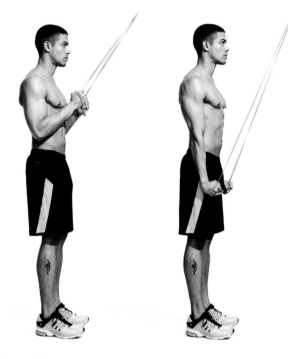

3B BICEPS CURL

SETS: 4 REPS: 15 REST: 60 SEC.

Anchor the band under your feet, holding an
end in each hand. Curl it without letting your
upper arms drift forward.

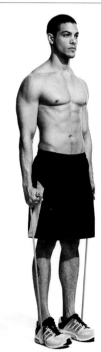
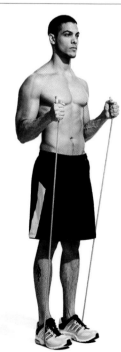

08 SUSPENSION TRAINER

The suspension trainer boom began about a decade ago, and what was once a piece of novel equipment is now hanging in gyms everywhere. The most popular brand, of course, is the TRX (*trx.com*), but competitors like the Jungle Gym XT (*lifelineusa.com*)—which we use to show the exercises that follow—are fine, too, so long as they offer foot cradles for performing lower-body exercises.

With a suspension trainer's incredible versatility, the number of exercises you can perform with it is about as limitless as your imagination. It allows you to train the whole body using exercises that would be nearly impossible with free weights, machines, or any other equipment. And unlike those other tools, the suspension trainer can travel anywhere you do, and takes up about as much space in your suitcase as a pair of pants.

We suggest you don't leave home without either one.

THE BEST SUSPENSION-TRAINER WORKOUT

WORKOUT #15   BY JAY CARDIELLO

A suspension trainer, such as the TRX or Jungle Gym XT, can mean the difference between sticking with your training while on the road and returning from your travels feeling slobbish. So long as your suspension trainer is fully adjustable and offers foot cradles you'll have a total-body gym that you can unpack from your suitcase whenever, wherever.

HOW IT WORKS The kind of instability a suspension trainer provides is ideal for core strengthening. To increase the instability, we've designed this workout using unilateral exercises, meaning that you'll be training each side of your body individually. If you need to reduce the intensity of an exercise, simply increase the angle of your body to the floor (shorten the length of the handles/straps).

The workout at right lets you customize your training, giving you a specific period of time in which to do your reps, rather than a concrete number of reps to hit every set.

DIRECTIONS Perform the exercises as a circuit, completing one set of each in sequence. Do as many reps as you can in 30 seconds, resting only as long as it takes to set up the next exercise. Perform two to four circuits.

1 SINGLE-LEG ROW

REPS: AS MANY AS POSSIBLE IN 30 SEC. (EACH SIDE) REST: 0 SEC.

Attach a suspension trainer to a doorframe or other sturdy object and stand on your left leg. Hold the handles and get into a lunge position with your rear knee bent—but keep your foot raised above the floor. Row your body to the handles while driving your right knee up in front of you.

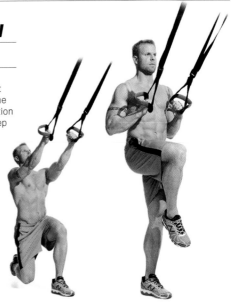

2 SINGLE-LEG WOBBLE LUNGE

REPS: AS MANY AS POSSIBLE IN 30 SEC. (EACH SIDE) REST: 0 SEC.

Set the foot cradle of the suspension trainer to about a foot and a half above the floor and turn around. Raise your right foot and rest it inside the cradle. Bend your left knee so you descend into a lunge position.

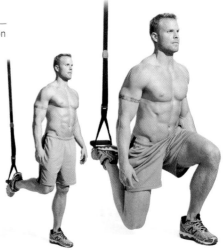

3 UNI-BRIDGE PRESS

REPS: AS MANY AS POSSIBLE IN
30 SEC. (EACH SIDE) REST: 0 SEC.

Face the suspension trainer's
attachment point and hold one
handle in your left hand. Pick up a
water bottle (or some other source
of light resistance) in your right hand
as if you were going to press. Lean
back so your body is in a straight
line at an angle, suspended by the
handle. Row your body up until
the handle touches your ribs
while pressing the right hand
over your chest.

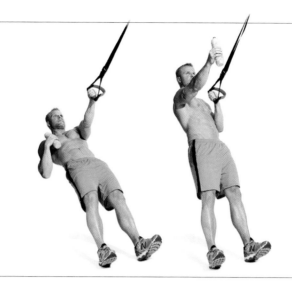

4 TAP OUT

REPS: AS MANY AS POSSIBLE IN
30 SEC. (EACH SIDE) REST: 0 SEC.

Set your feet in the cradles of the
trainer and get into pushup position.
Keeping your body straight, reach
up with your right hand and tap the
inside of your left elbow. Put your
hand back down and repeat with the
left hand. Continue for 30 seconds.

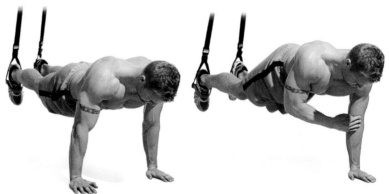

5 PUSHUP ROCKET

REPS: AS MANY AS POSSIBLE IN 30 SEC. REST: 0 SEC.

Get into pushup position with your feet in the cradles of the trainer and perform
explosive pushups so that your hands leave the floor and you can clap in midair.

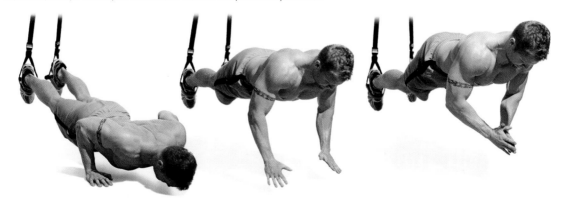

09

MEDICINE BALL

The first medicine balls, used by athletes in ancient Persia, were bladders filled with sand. While medicine ball construction has come a long way since then, the science of how to use one hasn't really had to evolve.

Med balls can be thrown, caught, rested on, or lifted like other weights, to apply a variety of stimuli to the muscles. Whether you want to experiment with one as a fun way to change up your workouts, or you find yourself someplace where the med ball (or a similar-sized volleyball or soccer ball) is the only implement you have to work with, we can show you how to use it like the sophisticated tool that it is.

THE BEST MEDICINE-BALL WORKOUT

WORKOUT #16   BY ZACH EVEN-ESH

The medicine ball has been around forever, but most guys don't know what to do with it, besides holding it against their chests during sit-ups. Even a light ball can deliver an intense workout that burns fat and builds athletic power.

HOW IT WORKS The med ball can be used to replicate various Olympic weightlifting exercises, and it makes performing them much simpler. These burn calories and build speed, which is helpful if you're interested in being competitive in backyard pickup games. In fact, the med ball is probably the most useful tool for developing explosive strength because it's meant to be thrown as hard as possible. When you toss it, you teach your body to accelerate without braking itself for safety.

Imagine a bench press done explosively–your shoulders must slow it down at the end of the range of motion or they risk getting torn out of their sockets by the speed. The ball allows your body to "let go" safely be-cause, well, you actually let go.

A med ball can also be used to create an unstable surface, such as by doing pushups on it. The dome shape forces you to stabilize your body more or risk taking a spill, and that means more activation of the abs.

DIRECTIONS Perform the exercise pairs (marked "A" and "B") as supersets, so you'll complete one set of A and then B before resting. Repeat until all sets are complete and then go on to the next superset.

1A CLEAN AND PRESS

SETS: 3 REPS: 10 REST: 0 SEC.

Hold the ball and stand with feet shoulder width. Bend your hips and knees and lower your body with arms extended until the ball is just above knee level. Explosively extend your hips and knees as if jumping, shrug your shoulders, and raise the ball to shoulder level. Squat down as you "catch" the momentum of the ball. Stand up and press it over-head. That's one rep.

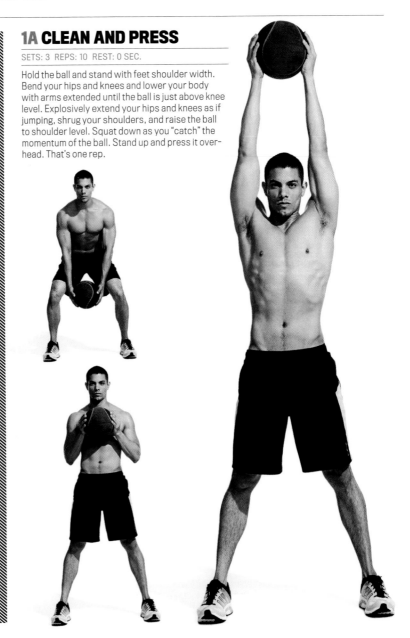

1B SITUP AND THROW

SETS: 3 REPS: 10 REST: 60 SEC.

Hold the ball with both hands in front of your chest and sit on the floor. Anchor your feet under something sturdy for support, and lie back on the floor a few feet away from a brick or concrete wall. Explosively sit up and throw the ball into the wall and then catch it on the rebound. If you have a partner, you can throw the ball to him instead and let him throw it back.

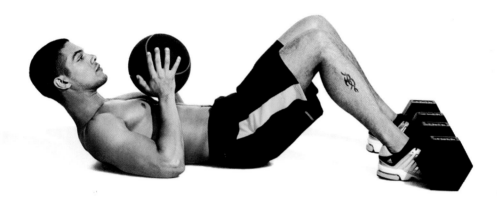

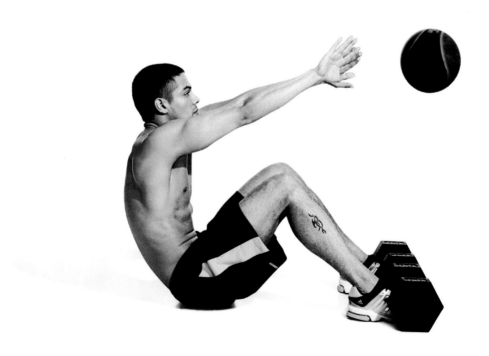

2A MOUNTAIN CLIMBER

SETS: 2 REPS: 20 (EACH LEG) REST: 0 SEC.

Hold the ball with both hands and get into pushup position on the floor. Drive one knee up to your chest and then quickly drive it back while you raise the opposite knee.

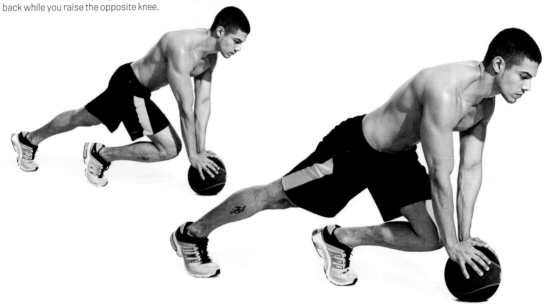

2B CLOSE-GRIP PUSHUP

SETS: 2 REPS: 15 REST: 60 SEC.

Get into pushup position on the floor, resting your hands on the ball. Keeping your body straight and your core braced, perform a pushup on the ball.

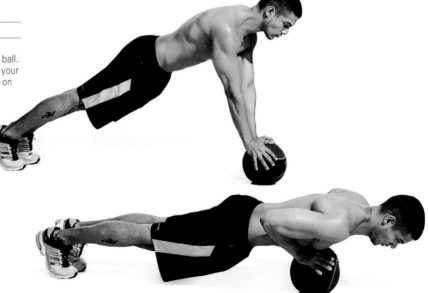

3A BULGARIAN SPLIT SQUAT

SETS: 2 REPS: 10 (EACH SIDE) REST: 0 SEC.

Stand lunge length in front of a bench holding the ball with both hands at arm's length overhead. Bend your left knee and rest the top of your left foot on the bench behind you. Lower your body until your front thigh is parallel to the floor.

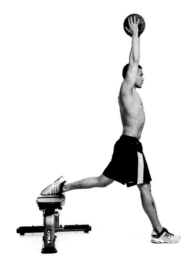
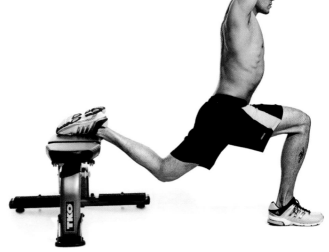

3B SEATED KNEE TUCK

SETS: 2 REPS: 10 REST: 60 SEC.

Sit on a bench and squeeze the ball between your feet. Extend and elevate your legs out in front of you and extend your torso so that your body forms a straight line. Hold on to the bench for support. Crunch your torso forward and bring your knees to your chest.

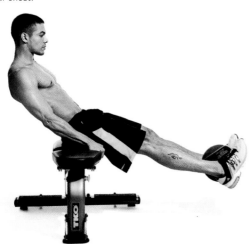
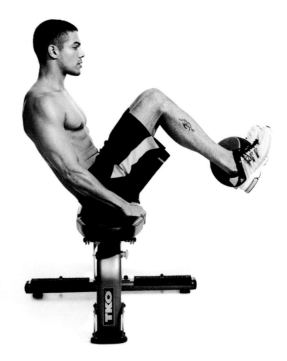

10

SWISS BALL

Swiss balls were created as a tool for rehab, but their value in working the core and a host of stabilizer muscles is now universally known. If you're a man of average height (about 5'9"), a ball with a 65-centimeter diameter will work best for you. Always make sure the ball is fully inflated and, for heaven's sake, don't try to stand on it. Wacky parlor tricks have given the Swiss ball a bad name, but used properly, it can improve your balance and strength rather than deprive you of them.

THE BEST SWISS-BALL WORKOUT

WORKOUT #17   BY JIM SMITH, C.S.C.S.

It may be hard to imagine working your entire body with just a Swiss ball. After all, you can't curl it, press it, or squat it. But the ball can let you get into positions to work your muscles that you wouldn't normally think of, and the stability those positions require works more muscle than you realize.

HOW IT WORKS Many of the exercises flow into each other or consist of combinations of movements that flow together to equal one rep. Controlling these movements on an unstable ball makes every move a core exercise, even while you're targeting the chest, shoulders, legs, and back.

DIRECTIONS Perform the exercises as a circuit, completing one set of each in turn without rest. After the last exercise, rest two to three minutes and then repeat the entire circuit for three total sets.

1 PUSHUP W/ FEET ON BALL

SETS: 3 REPS: 20 REST: 0 SEC.

Get into pushup position on the floor with hands shoulder width and rest your feet on the ball. Brace your abs and lower your body until your chest is just above the floor. Push back up. Do not let your hips dip or sway side to side at any point.

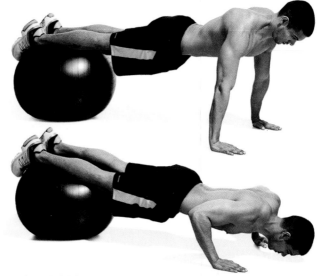

2 T ON BALL

SETS: 3 REPS: 20 REST: 0 SEC.

Lie chest-down on the ball and raise your arms out in front of you with palms facing up. Now move them out 90 degrees to form a T shape. Hold for one or two seconds with your shoulder blades squeezed together.

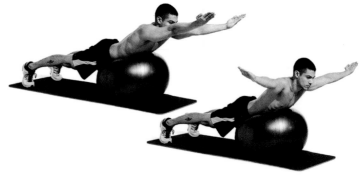

3 BODY-WEIGHT SQUAT

SETS: 3 REPS: 20 REST: 0 SEC.

Stand with feet shoulder width and toes turned out slightly. Sit back with your hips and lower your body as far as you can without rounding your lower back. Push your knees out as you descend and keep your chest up.

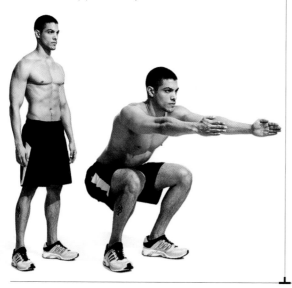

4 LEG CURL

SETS: 3 REPS: 20 REST: 0 SEC.

Lie on your back on the floor and rest your heels on a Swiss ball. Brace your abs and drive your heels into the ball to raise your hips off the floor. Bend your knees and roll the ball toward you. Keep your hips elevated the entire set.

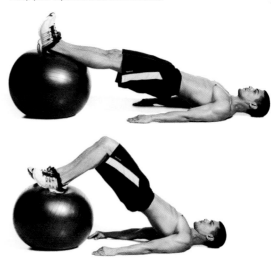

5 PIKE-UP TO SUPERMAN

SETS: 3 REPS: 20 REST: 120–180 SEC.

Get into pushup position with your toes on the ball. Bend your hips and roll the ball toward you so your torso becomes vertical. Roll back so your body is straight again and extend your spine, then roll the ball up your legs so your body forms a straight line with arms extended overhead but hands still on the floor. You should look like Superman flying downward. That's one rep. Pull with your lats to return to the pushup position and begin the next rep.

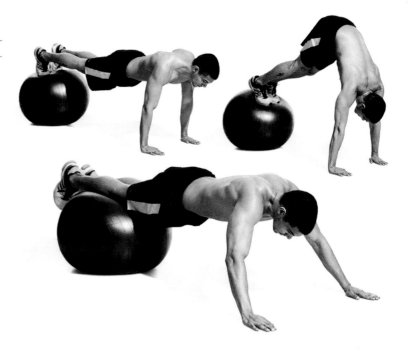

11 BODY WEIGHT

The most obvious advantage of body-weight workouts is that you can do them without equipment and in almost any location. But if that means absolutely no equipment—as in, not even a pullup bar—you'll need to get pretty creative to be able to work your back.

We got that creative.

When it's warm, you may want to take your workouts outdoors and make use of equipment at your local playground, but you may not know how best to make a workout with it.

We know how to make a workout with it.

If you thought body-weight training was just pushups and situps, these routines will open your eyes to the multitude of ways you can get ripped at those times when you feel as if you have no options at all.

THE BEST
BODY-WEIGHT WORKOUT [option A]

WORKOUT #18   BY ZACH EVEN-ESH

If you've ever wondered how guys who work out exclusively on monkey bars in the park get so ripped, this workout is the answer. We hope you'll take it outside on a summer day, but it can work just as well in a bare-bones garage gym. Not only will you burn fat and build muscle with just three exercises—you'll learn one of the secrets street gymnasts use to bang out dozens of reps of pullups and dips at a clip: the 10 to 1 method.

HOW IT WORKS The circuit we've designed here doesn't let up. When you train any squat variation, plus the pullup and the dip, you work nearly every muscle in your body, and your heart will race to supply them with blood and oxygen. Performing a decreasing number of reps—10 to 1—helps you keep the workout going despite being fatigued and builds the endurance that ultimately leads to being able to rattle off a high number of reps in one shot. In addition to getting you leaner, feel free to use this workout to win bar bets about how many pullups you can do.

DIRECTIONS Perform the exercises as a circuit, completing a set of each in turn and resting as little as possible between sets. Repeat for 10 circuits (until you're doing only one rep per exercise).

1 JUMP SQUAT

REPS: 10 TO 1 REST: 0 SEC.

Stand with feet shoulder-width apart and squat down about halfway. Jump as high as you can. Land with soft knees and begin the next rep. Perform 10 reps. Each time you repeat the circuit, perform one less rep. So the next round you'll do 9 reps, then 8, and so on down to 1 rep.

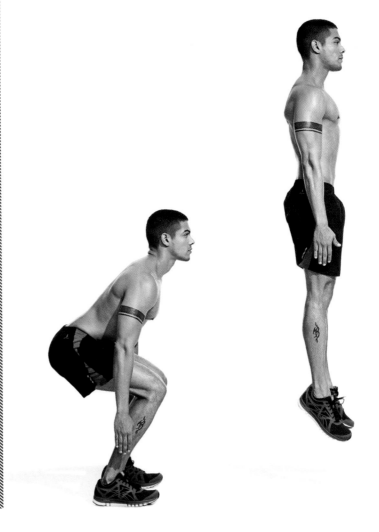

2 PULLUP

REPS: 10 TO 1 REST: 0 SEC.

Hang from a pullup bar, jungle gym, or tree limb and pull yourself up until your chin is higher than your hands. Perform 10 reps down to 1 as described at left.

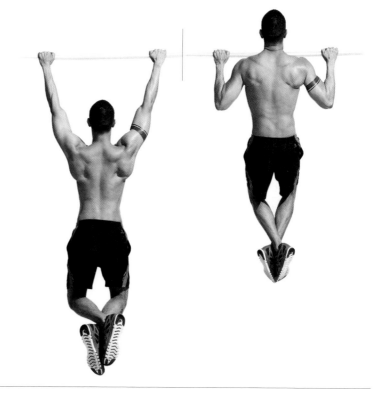

3 DIP

REPS: 10 TO 1 REST: 0 SEC.

Suspend yourself over parallel bars and then lower your body until your upper arms are parallel to the floor. Perform 10 reps down to 1.

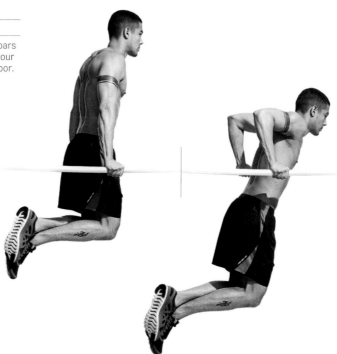

THE BEST BODY-WEIGHT WORKOUT [option B]

WORKOUT #19   BY ZACH EVEN-ESH

A lack of training equipment doesn't necessarily doom you to a workout consisting only of pullups and pushups. With a little creativity, you can still train like an animal (you'll get the reference below) while targeting your entire body—not just the upper. This workout is outside the box—so much so, in fact, that you'll have to go outdoors to do it.

HOW IT WORKS This routine requires a park or playground area with monkey bars and plenty of open space. You'll use classic, though under-prescribed, body-weight exercises like the bear crawl and crab walk, which you probably haven't tried since your days in summer camp. As you'll come to remember, they're not easy—especially for a grown man well north of 100 pounds. They require a lot of work from your heart, lungs, and core. Later, the parallel bar hand walk will blow up your grip and forearms; the sprints will fry your legs.

DIRECTIONS Perform the exercise pairs (marked "A" and "B") as supersets, so you'll complete one set of A and then one set of B before resting. Repeat until all sets are complete. Note that the parallel bar hand walk is done as straight sets—do a set, rest, and repeat.

This workout combines well with Body-Weight option A, so if you want to integrate them both into a training week, perform A first, rest a day, and then perform B. (You can also add in option C, coming up next.)

1A BEAR CRAWL

SETS: 3 REPS: CRAWL FOR 50 FEET REST: 0 SEC.

Bend down and plant your hands on the ground. Try to keep your back flat as you walk on all fours as fast as you can. Your legs should be fairly straight as you step your feet outside where your hands land.

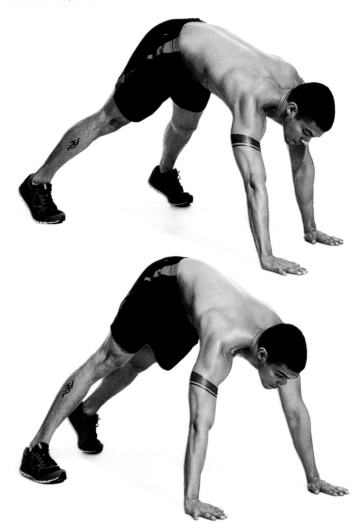

1B CRAB WALK

SETS: 3 REPS: WALK FOR 50 FEET REST: AS NEEDED

Sit on the ground and bridge up with your hips so you look like a tabletop. Walk forward on your hands and feet as fast as you can.

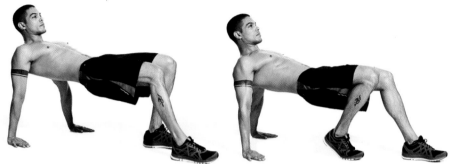

2 PARALLEL BAR HAND WALK

SETS: 5 REPS: WALK TO THE END AND BACK REST: AS NEEDED

Hang from a jungle gym or length of parallel bars. Walk to the end of the row and back with your hands.

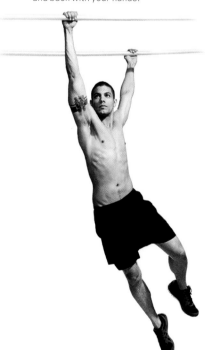

3A FORWARD SPRINT

SETS: 5 REPS: SPRINT 50 YARDS
REST: 0 SEC.

Run at about 90% of your top speed.

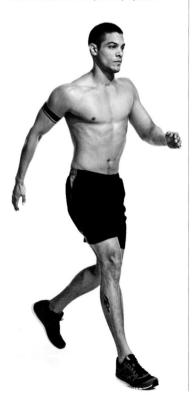

3B BACKWARD SPRINT

SETS: 5 REPS: SPRINT 50 YARDS
REST: AS NEEDED

Run backward as quickly as you can.

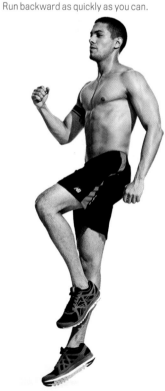

THE BEST
BODY-WEIGHT WORKOUT [option C]

WORKOUT #20   BY ZACH EVEN-ESH

Combining exercises whenever possible helps you work more muscles in the same amount of time. These hybrid moves allow you to get the benefit of six exercises in a workout that actually prescribes only three.

HOW IT WORKS This workout can be combined with the previous two for a three-day-per-week program done in the order shown. Or, combine it with either one of the two previous workouts and alternate them throughout the week.

DIRECTIONS Perform the exercises as conventional straight sets, completing all sets for one exercise before moving on to the next. If you can't perform 10 reps for a particular set, do as many as you can without going to failure (end the set with one or two reps in you) and then rest a few moments. Continue when you can to complete the remaining reps.

1 BURPEE TO BROAD JUMP

SETS: 3 REPS: 10 REST: 90 SEC.

Bend down and place your hands on the floor. Now shoot your legs behind you fast so you end up in the top of a pushup position. Perform a pushup and then jump your legs back up to your hands. From there, jump forward as far as you can.

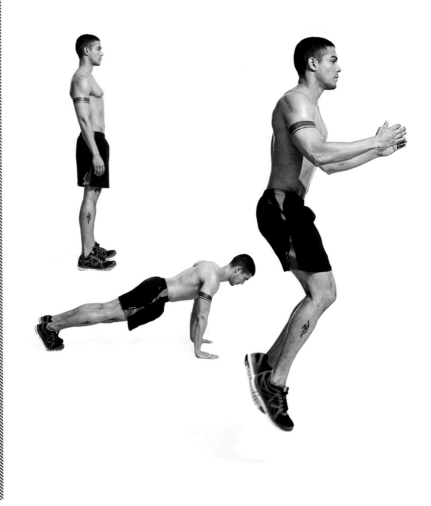

2 DIP TO LEG RAISE

SETS: 3 REPS: 10

Suspend your body over parallel bars
and lower yourself until your upper
arms are parallel to the floor. Press
yourself back up and then raise your
legs straight out in front of you.

3 PULLUP TO KNEE RAISE

SETS: 3 REPS: 10

Hang from a pullup bar with hands
outside shoulder width and palms
facing away from you. Pull yourself
up until your chin is over the bar and
then raise your knees to your chest in
the top position.

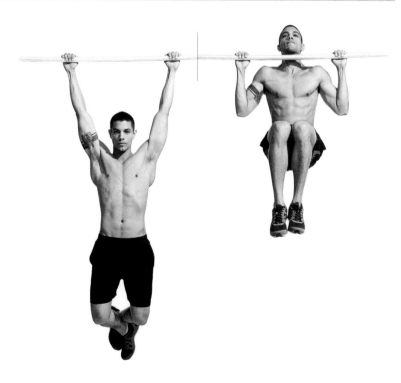

THE BEST
BODY-WEIGHT WORKOUT [option D]

WORKOUT #21   BY JOE STANKOWSKI, C.P.T.

OK, we'll admit it: Sometimes the odds really are against your getting a workout in. You may well find yourself stuck without weights or bands, only to find that you also forgot to pack your suspension trainer. There's nothing to pull on, so you can't work your back, and you can't even improvise with the objects around you.

We're not sure just what kind of place this would be, short of a jail cell (and if that's where you are, hey, we're not judging), but we can give you a great workout to do, even there.

HOW IT WORKS All you need is something to step on, be it a park bench, a large rock, or a chair. But if you have nothing elevated on which to step, you can substitute a lunge for the stepup. To target your back, which is usually unworkable without having at least a bar of some sort to pull on, we're employing the "blurpee"–as made famous by fitness expert Tim Ferriss, author of *The Four-Hour Body.*

The wider foot placement used in the blurpee requires more work from the lats to pull the hips and legs forward as the body comes back from the pushup position. (The extra "l" in blurpee stands for "lats.")

DIRECTIONS Perform the exercises as conventional straight sets, completing all sets for one exercise before moving on to the next.

1 CLOSE-GRIP PUSHUP

SETS: 3 REPS: 15 REST: 60-90 SEC.

Get into pushup position and place your hands close so that your thumbs touch. Keep your body straight and your core braced. If that's too easy, elevate your feet on a chair or some other raised surface.

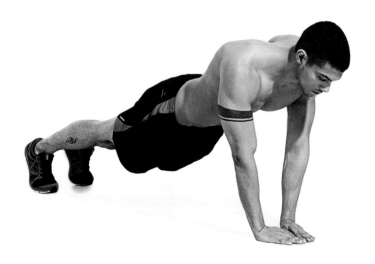

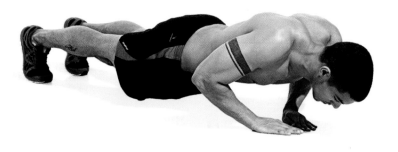

2 STEPUP

SETS: 3 REPS: 20 REST: 60-90 SEC.

Stand in front of a bench or chair and place one foot on it so that your thigh is parallel to the floor. Drive your heel into the surface and squeeze your glutes as you step up onto the bench, but let your trailing foot hang off of it.

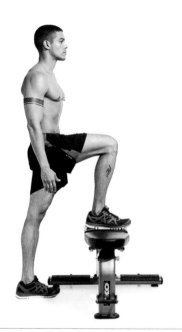
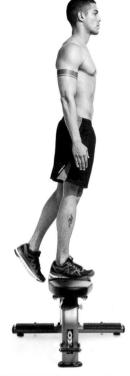

3 BLURPEE

SETS: 3 REPS: 20 REST: 60-90 SEC.

Stand with feet outside shoulder width and bend down and place your hands on the floor. Now shoot your legs behind you fast so you end up in the top of a pushup position. Jump your legs back up so they land to the outside of your hands and then jump up quickly.

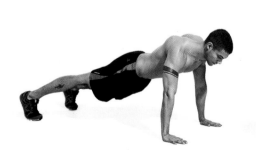
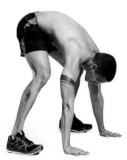
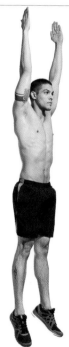

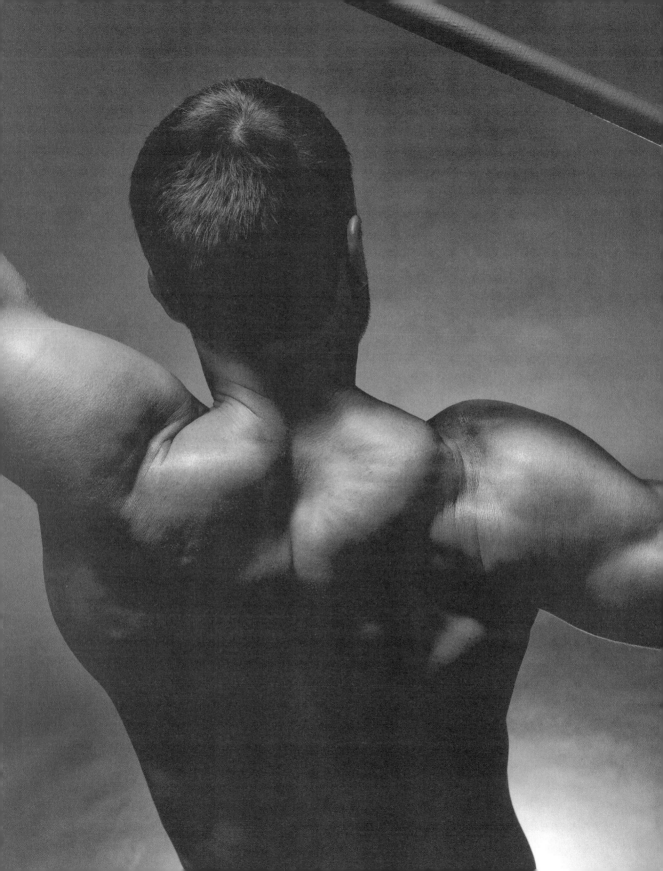

BODY PART WORKOUTS

12

ARMS

Since it's likely that arms were your first priority when you began training, and will continue to be for the rest of your life, we put this body part first. Not that you'll ever get bored of bombing your bi's and tri's, but we've provided you with five different ways to work them—with a barbell, dumbbells, bands, a suspension trainer, and yes, even body weight alone. Just try to leave some time in your week for the leg workouts, OK?

THE BEST DUMBBELL-ONLY ARM WORKOUT

WORKOUT #22   BY JIM SMITH, C.S.C.S.

You can't go wrong with a pair of dumbbells. Arguably the most versatile equipment in a trainer's arsenal, dumbbells are a favorite among competitive bodybuilders, who happen to know a thing or two about stacking impressive arms. Whether or not you want bodybuild-eresque arms, dumbbells can prove invaluable in your quest to improve them.

HOW IT WORKS You'll make use of peak contractions (holding the top, flexed, position of a rep for a second or two), slow negatives (lowering the weight with control), and stretching between sets. All of these strategies increase blood flow to the arms and encourage growth.

DIRECTIONS Perform 1A and 1B as supersets. So you'll complete one set of A and then go on to B before resting. Repeat for the prescribed sets. Exercises 2A, 2B, and 2C are a triset—complete one set of each without rest and then repeat for all the prescribed sets.

1A SEATED CURL

SETS: 3 REPS: 12 REST: 0 SEC.

Sit on an incline bench or seat with a backrest holding a dumbbell in each hand. Keeping your upper arms against your sides, curl the weights simultaneously, rotating your wrists outward so that your palms face you in the top position. Hold the top position for two seconds, squeezing your biceps, and take three to five seconds to lower the weights on each rep.

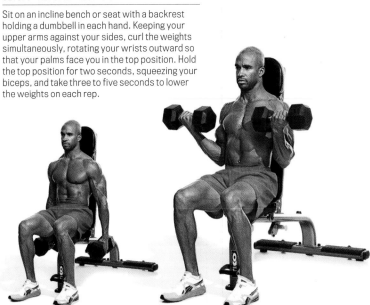

1B DIAMOND PUSHUP

SETS: 3 REPS: 20 REST: 60 SEC.

Get into pushup position but place your hands close together so your thumbs and index fingers touch. Keeping your body in a straight line with abs braced, lower your torso until your chest is just above the floor and then press back up.

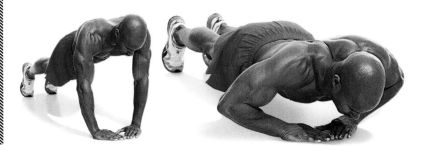

2A HAMMER CURL

SETS: 4 REPS: 8 REST: 0 SEC.

Hold a dumbbell in each hand with palms facing your sides. Keeping your upper arms against your sides, curl the weights at the same time.

2B NEUTRAL-GRIP TRICEPS EXTENSION

SETS: 4 REPS: 12 REST: 0 SEC.

Lie back on a bench or the floor holding a dumbbell in each hand with palms facing each other. Press the weights over your chest and then bend your elbows to lower the weights toward your face until you feel a stretch in your triceps. Extend your elbows. Keep your elbows facing the ceiling the entire set.

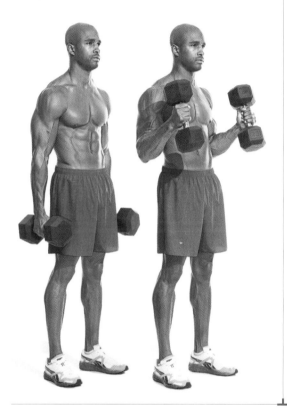

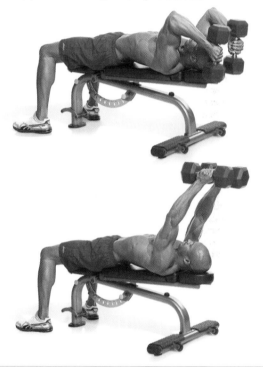

2C BICEPS/TRICEPS STRETCH

SETS: 4 REPS: HOLD FOR 30 SEC. (EACH SIDE)

Place the palm of one hand on a bench, box, or other low, flat surface with your fingers pointing toward you. Lean away to apply a stretch and hold it for 30 seconds. Now reach your arm overhead and bend the elbow. Gently pull your arm behind your head to stretch your triceps for 30 seconds.

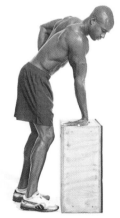

THE BEST BARBELL-ONLY ARM WORKOUT

WORKOUT #23   BY JASON FERRUGGIA

A barbell's main selling point is that it allows you to maximally stimulate muscle, but it isn't written in stone (or, perhaps, iron) that you must use heavy weights, or any weight at all. If a barbell is all you have to train with, we'll assume that you don't have a lot of weight at your disposal anyway, so this workout is a minimalist's dream.

HOW IT WORKS The Poundstone curl is simply a barbell curl done with the empty bar alone–for an enormous number of reps (in this case, we prescribe 100). It's named after professional strongman Derek Poundstone, who, despite being 350 pounds with biceps like footballs, still swears by this deceptively hard exercise. The point is simply to give the biceps shock treatment with a protocol they've never encountered before–very high reps and short rest until exhaustion.

The pullover/triceps extension works your lats as well as your triceps. By getting the lats involved, you incorporate strong stabilizing muscles that will let you go a little heavier on the triceps extensions–even if all the weight you have left to add is a couple of 2.5-pound plates.

DIRECTIONS Perform all the sets for the first exercise before moving on to the second.

1 POUNDSTONE CURL

SETS: AS MANY AS NEEDED   REPS: 100 TOTAL   REST: AS NEEDED

Grasp the barbell at shoulder width. Keeping your upper arms at your sides, curl the bar.

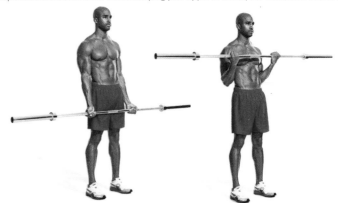

2 PULLOVER/TRICEPS EXTENSION

SETS: 6   REPS: 12-15   REST: 45 SEC.

Hold the bar with an overhand, shoulder-width grip and lie back on a flat bench. Press the bar toward the ceiling and then reach it back over your head while bending your elbows until you feel a stretch in your lats. Then pull the bar back over your chest and extend your elbows.

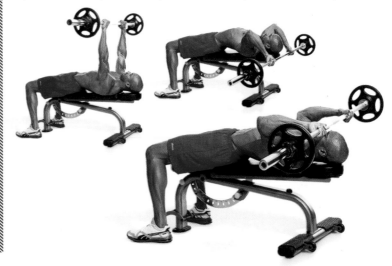

THE BEST BAND-ONLY ARM WORKOUT

WORKOUT #24   BY NICK TUMMINELLO

Sometimes building muscle is as simple as doing reps as fast as you can to get a pump as quickly as possible. It may sound haphazard, but this band-only workout can add as much as an inch to your upper arms in just six weeks!

HOW IT WORKS This workout should be implemented for a period of six weeks—enough time to elicit growth, but not so much as to allow your muscles to adapt to the stresses. Over this time period, you'll gradually increase the volume you perform on your exercises (there are only two), which forces your body to adapt to a rapidly increasing workload. The pushdown and curl pump your arms full of blood, driving nutrients into the muscles and stretching their cells. As fun as the pump is for showing off, it's also a sign that real growth is on the way.

DIRECTIONS Alternate the band pushdown and band curl. Perform each move twice. If you like, repeat the workout once per week for up to six weeks. Perform two sets the second week as well, followed by three sets in Weeks 3 and 4. In Weeks 5 and 6, perform four sets. Assuming you're following the weight-gain eating rules outlined in Chapter 1, you could see up to a solid inch added to your arms in that span.

1 BAND PUSHDOWN

REPS: 60   REST: 0 SEC.

Attach the band to the top of a sturdy object, such as a pipe or a beam. If you're using a loop band, grasp the middle of it with both hands. Tuck your elbows to your sides and extend your elbows as in a triceps pushdown. Try to get 60 reps in 30 seconds. It's OK if you rock back and forth a bit.

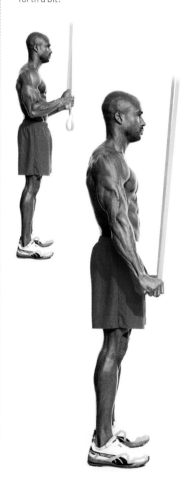

2 BAND CURL

REPS: 60   REST: 120 SEC.

Anchor the band under your feet, holding the other end with both hands. Curl as fast as you can for 30 seconds, aiming again for 60 reps.

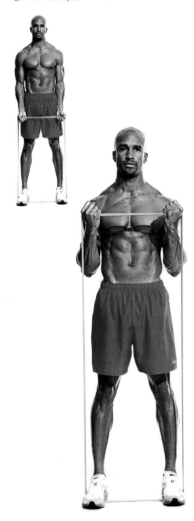

THE BEST SUSPENSION-TRAINER ARM WORKOUT

WORKOUT #25   BY BEN BRUNO

Over the past decade, suspension trainers have skyrocketed in popularity, and for good reason. The kind of whole-body training you can perform on a suspension system is as efficient as it is effective, and studies have shown that compound movements release more muscle-building hormones than do isolation moves. While the following workout seems to target your entire upper body, the stress it places on your arms in particular will get them looking as good as if they were trained with isolation movements.

HOW IT WORKS The workout starts with pushups and rows. It will hit the chest, shoulders, and back, too, of course; but it won't shortchange your biceps and triceps. In fact, even though you're not working them in isolation, the bi's and tri's will kick in harder because they're lifting more of your weight than they could if you were doing simple curls or extensions. Nevertheless, there's a place for these movements, too—right after the compound lifts, when you're looking to finish the arms off with more direct stimulation.

DIRECTIONS Perform the exercise pairs (marked "A" and "B") as alternating sets. You'll do a set of A, rest, then a set of B, rest again, and continue for all the prescribed sets.

1A PUSHUP

SETS: 4   REPS: 10–12   REST: 60 SEC.

Attach the suspension trainer to a sturdy overhead object and lengthen the straps to a point where you're sure you can do 10–12 pushups. (You can lower the handles over time to make the set harder, and later, elevate your feet; shorten the straps to make it easier.) Grasp the handles and get into pushup position with hands under your shoulders. Your entire body should be straight and your core braced. Lower your body until your chest is between the handles.

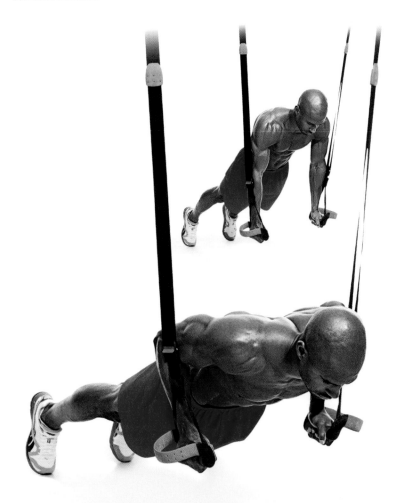

1B ROTATIONAL INVERTED ROW

SETS: 4   REPS: 10-12   REST: 60 SEC.

Hold the handles and lean back with arms extended so that your body is supported by the trainer and only your feet are on the floor. Brace your core and hold your body in a straight line. (The lower you set the handles, the harder the exercise; you can elevate your feet to make it even harder.) Start with your palms facing your feet, and as you row your body up, twist your wrists outward so that your palms face up in the top position.

2A TRICEPS EXTENSION

SETS: 4   REPS: 10   REST: 60 SEC.

Lengthen the straps and stand underneath the trainer's anchor point. Lean your weight forward and bend your elbows so you feel a stretch in your triceps. Your palms should face each other behind your head. Keeping your body straight and your abs braced, extend your elbows, rotating your palms so they face down in the extended position.

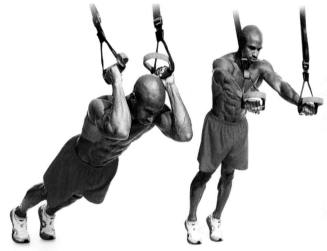

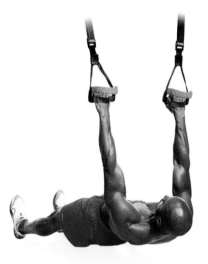

2B BICEPS CURL

SETS: 4   REPS: 10   REST: 60 SEC.

Face the trainer's attachment point and grasp the handles with palms facing up. Lean back with your abs braced, body straight, and arms extended in front of you. Curl your body up to the handles.

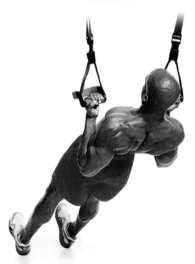

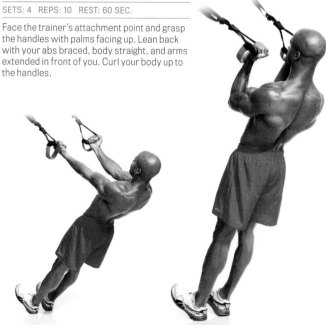

THE BEST
BODY-WEIGHT ARM WORKOUT

WORKOUT #26   BY BEN BRUNO

What if you've got nothing—no barbells, no dumbbells, no bands, or a suspension system—but are still itching to pump up the guns? No problem! So long as you can find an overhead pipe or crossbar that will support your weight, and some level ground, you can work your arms. In fact, by following the workout below, you won't just work your arms; you'll make them grow.

HOW IT WORKS Upper-body training, in its simplest terms, is about pushing and pulling. Pair the two movement patterns up and you've got a complete arm blast, and that's what we did here. You'll finish with eccentric chinups, which are just normal chins done with an extra-slow negative. This causes more muscle damage in the biceps, leading to greater growth, and that's always cool—even if there's no one else around to notice.

DIRECTIONS Perform the exercise pairs (marked "A" and "B") as alternating sets. You'll do a set of A, rest, then a set of B, rest again, and continue for all the prescribed sets.

1A CLOSE-GRIP PUSHUP

SETS: 5   REPS: 12–15   REST: 60 SEC.

Place your hands inside shoulder width and lower your body until your chest is about an inch above the floor. To increase the difficulty, elevate your feet on a bench or box.

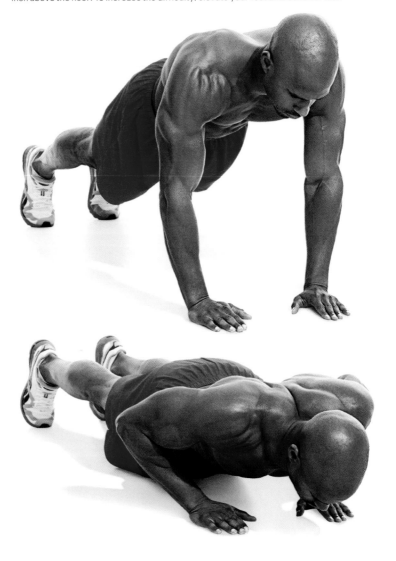

1B CHINUP

SETS: 5   REPS: 6–8   REST: 60 SEC.

Grasp the chinup bar at (or slightly inside) shoulder width, with palms facing you. Pull yourself up until your chin is over the bar.

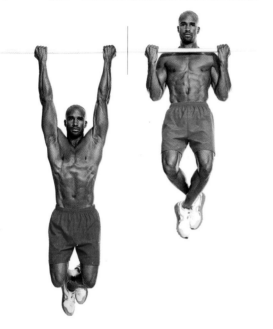

2A TRICEPS EXTENSION

SETS: 4   REPS: 10   REST: 60 SEC.

Get into pushup position and rest your forearms on the floor, palms down. Keeping your core tight and your body in a straight line, extend your elbows so your arms are straight.

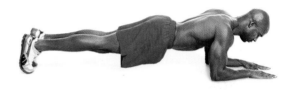

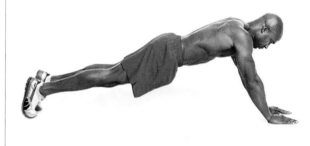

2B ECCENTRIC CHINUP

SETS: 4   REPS: 3   REST: 60 SEC.

Grasp a chinup bar at shoulder width with palms facing you and jump into the top position of a chinup. Take five seconds to lower yourself down to the hang position. That's one rep.

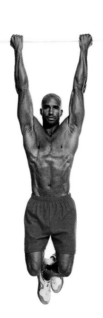

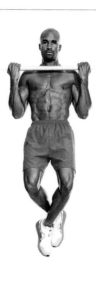

13

BICEPS

When you first start training, an equal amount of arm work for the biceps and triceps is enough to stimulate even gains. But down the line, one muscle always seems to develop ahead of the other and you end up needing to give the weaker one greater attention. If it's your biceps, you're about to learn a bevy of new curls that will peak your peaks fast and for a long time to come.

THE BEST
FULL-GYM BICEPS WORKOUT

WORKOUT #27   BY HARRY CLAY

When you've got total gym access you need to take advantage of it. However, for the more zealous among us, there is a risk of overtraining smaller body parts–like biceps–in an attempt to sample all of a gym's wares. That's why you'll want to keep overall volume low for biceps, in comparison with bigger body parts, like back and chest. The following workout provides good variety and intensity while avoiding the common pitfall of overtraining.

HOW IT WORKS You won't be doing a lot of work, but every exercise was carefully chosen. Fattening the grip on dumbbell curls requires more tension from your hands and forearms to hoist the weight, and this transfers to your biceps. The rarely seen behind-the-back cable curl puts the biceps at an especially tough mechanical disadvantage, which forces you to overcome a lot of resistance as you contract them from a stretched position. The EZ-bar preacher curl finishes the workout with the strictest possible movement.

DIRECTIONS Perform the exercises at the end of an upper-body workout once per week.

1 FAT-GRIP HAMMER CURL

SETS: 3   REPS: 10-12   REST: 60 SEC.

Select two dumbbells and wrap towels around each handle to thicken it. Another option is to use rubber-grip sleeves like Fat Gripz (available at *fatgripz.com*) or Grip4orce (shown below, *grip4orce.com*). Keeping your upper arms stationary at your sides and your palms facing, curl the weights.

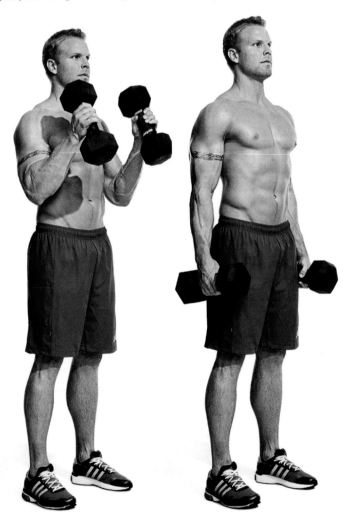

2 BEHIND-THE-BACK CABLE CURL

SETS: 3   REPS: 10-12 (EACH SIDE)
REST: 60 SEC.

Attach a D-handle to the low pulley of a cable machine, grasp the handle in your left hand, and step forward (away from the machine) until there is tension on the cable and your arm is drawn slightly behind your body. Stagger your feet so your right leg is in front. Curl the handle but do not allow your elbow to point forward.

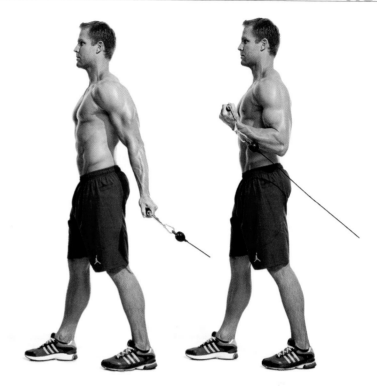

3 EZ-BAR PREACHER CURL

SETS: 2   REPS: 8-10   REST: 60 SEC.

Sit at a preacher bench and adjust the height so that your armpits touch the top of the bench. Grasp an EZ-curl bar at shoulder width with arms extended (but allow a slight bend at the elbows). Curl the bar, keeping the backs of your arms against the bench. Take three seconds to lower the bar back down.

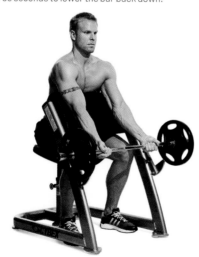

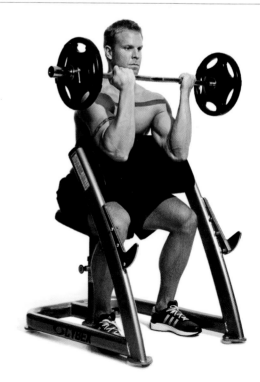

THE BEST BARBELL-ONLY BICEPS WORKOUT

WORKOUT #28   BY JIM SMITH, C.S.C.S.

The biceps are small muscles that aren't designed to handle a lot of weight, but they do respond well to high reps, short rest periods, and multiple angles. With only a barbell loaded with a modest amount of weight and some earnest effort, you can build a solid pair of biceps muscles without overtaxing your biceps tendons.

HOW IT WORKS The workout starts with a reverse curl–the weakest grip you can curl with because your palms are facing down. It gradually progresses you to curls in stronger positions so that you can use the heaviest weights possible and keep your intensity up even as fatigue sets in. And "fatigue" is putting it mildly. Twenty reps per set will have your arms in agony, and then you'll finish them with ladder sets–conventional curls done for more reps in each successive set until you're doing 50 with just the bar. By that point, that's all the weight you'll be able to lift.

DIRECTIONS Complete each exercise in turn. Hold the top of each repetition for one second and take two or three seconds to lower each rep.

1 REVERSE CURL

SETS: 1   REPS: 20   REST: 60 SEC.

Grasp the bar overhand at whatever width is comfortable. Keeping your upper arms against your sides, curl the bar.

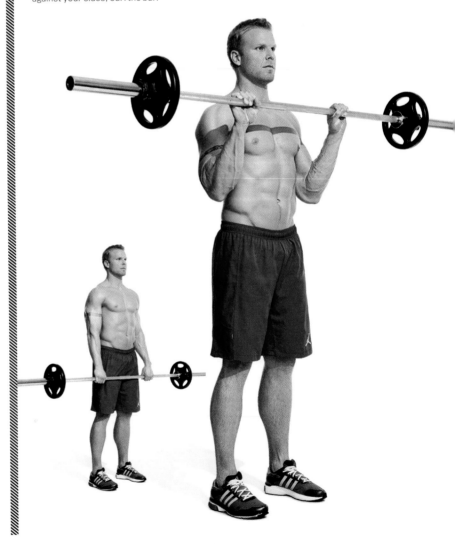

2 WIDE-GRIP CURL

SETS: 1 REPS: 20 REST: 60 SEC.

Grasp the bar with hands wider than shoulder width—if you're using an Olympic bar, your pinkies should be on the outside knurling. Perform curls.

3 CLOSE-GRIP CURL

SETS: 1 REPS: 20 REST: 60 SEC.

Curl with your hands inside shoulder width, in the middle of the bar.

4 CONVENTIONAL CURL

SETS: 4 REPS: 20, 30, 40, 50 REST: 60 SEC.

Place three 5-pound plates on each side of the bar, hands at shoulder width, and perform 20 reps. That's one set. Then take off one plate from each side. Perform 30 reps. Unload another plate from each side and do 40 reps. Finally, remove the last set of plates and do 50 reps with just the empty bar.

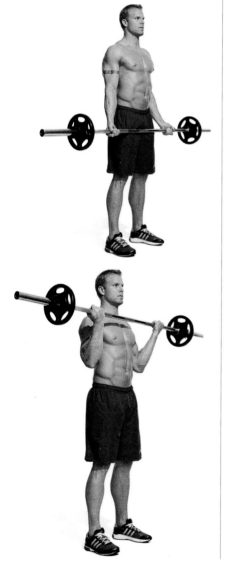

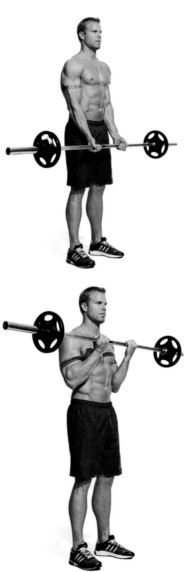

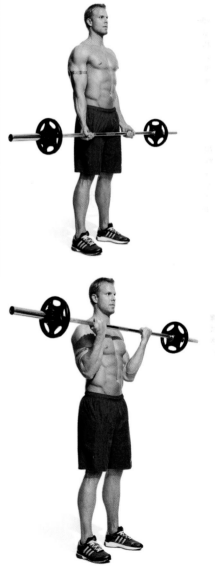

THE BEST DUMBBELL-ONLY BICEPS WORKOUT

WORKOUT #29   BY C.J. MURPHY, M.F.S.

You might think that cheating on an exercise is only cheating your muscles out of the best possible stimulus, but then how do you explain all the guys with mountainous biceps slinging dumbbells to their shoulders on curls? While we wouldn't recommend making bad form a staple in your workouts, we'll admit that sometimes it helps to break the rules, and with this dumbbell-only routine, we'll teach you how to cheat to win.

HOW IT WORKS The workout starts with strict dumbbell curls. Since you'll be fresh, you should have no trouble giving each set your utmost focus, using only the strength in your biceps to complete your reps. The drag curl follows—another movement that relies on precise form and prevents your shoulders or back from assisting. Later, you can loosen up, doing curls again but this time with intentional cheating. At this point, you'll be tired and unable to execute reps with perfect technique anyway, so you'll get a little help from your hips to power through your sticking point. Your biceps will still be working hard, and with most of your workout accomplished, all you need do now is top them off with blood to ensure the greatest growth.

DIRECTIONS Complete all the prescribed sets for one exercise before moving on to the next.

1 CURL

SETS: 4   REPS: 15, 12, 8, 8   REST: 60 SEC.

Stand holding a dumbbell in each hand with palms facing your sides. Keep your weight on your heels and lean forward slightly. Without letting your upper arms drift forward, curl the weights, rotating your wrists outward so that your palms face you in the top position. Hold the top for a moment and squeeze your biceps. Lower the weights back down and flex your triceps hard in the bottom position (your arms should end up slightly behind your body). Increase the weight gradually each set.

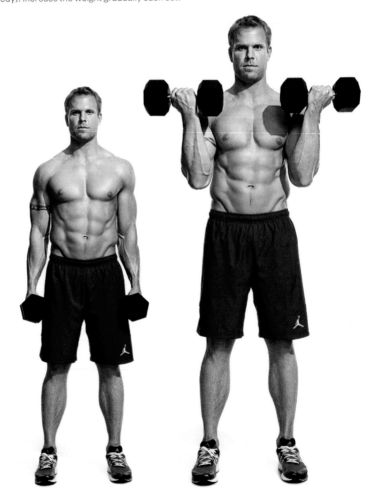

2 DRAG CURL

SETS: 4   REPS: 12–15   REST: 60 SEC.

Perform as you would the conventional dumbbell curl, but stand tall and drive your elbows back as you curl so the head of each dumbbell touches the front of your body throughout the rep. (Keep your palms facing up the whole time.) It should look as though you're dragging the weights up along your torso.

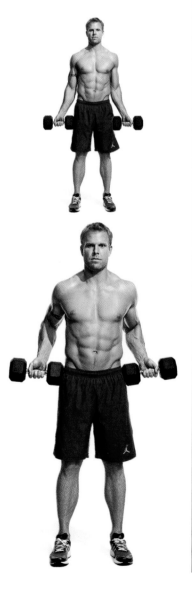

3 HAMMER CURL

SETS: 4   REPS: 15–20   REST: 60 SEC.

Perform as you did the conventional dumbbell curl but keep your palms facing your sides throughout.

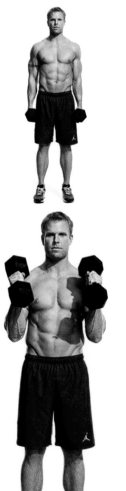

4 CHEAT CURL

SETS: 3   REPS: SEE BELOW   REST: 60 SEC.

Choose the heaviest dumbbells you think you can curl, and perform as you did the conventional dumbbell curl, but use momentum from your hips to power through the sticking point (halfway up, when the weights are most difficult to lift). Do not lean back as you lift, but get into a rhythm where you rock your torso forward and then extend your hips to complete each rep. Stop each set one rep shy of total failure.

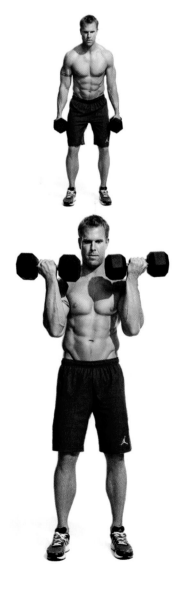

THE BEST
BAND-ONLY BICEPS WORKOUT

WORKOUT #30   BY C.J. MURPHY, M.F.S.

It was once thought that the pump was just a cosmetic side effect of lifting weights, but it's actually an integral part of the muscle-building process. Performing reps creates tension in the muscles that, to some degree, pinches off the veins that take blood out of them while the arteries that deliver blood to the muscles continue unobstructed. So the muscles fill up with blood faster than they can be cleared of it. This "cell swelling" stretches the muscle cell membranes, sending the body the message that the muscles aren't big enough to handle the blood flow to them.

Bands create enormous tension throughout a muscle's entire range of motion, and yet the tension is easily adjusted depending on how you stand or position your body. This makes them great tools for pumping up your biceps.

HOW IT WORKS The workout is designed for use with two or more bands, but if you have only one, you can perform any of the curls one arm at a time. On the high-rep, high-speed curls, keep your stance narrow (inside shoulder width) and adjust it as necessary to complete all your reps in one set.

DIRECTIONS Complete all the prescribed sets for one exercise before moving on to the next.

1 HIGH-SPEED CURL

SETS: AS MANY AS NEEDED   REPS: 100   REST: 60 SEC.

Anchor the band under your feet, holding the ends with both hands at your sides. Resist your elbows moving forward as you perform curls as fast as you can. Keep your body still.

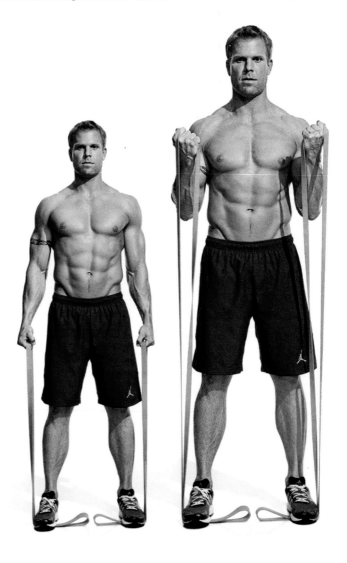

2 SIDE CURL

SETS: 4   REPS: 15-20   REST: 60 SEC.

Attach two bands to sturdy objects at shoulder
height that face each other. Stand between them and
hold an end in each hand. Raise your arms out 90
degrees with elbows extended—you should still feel
some tension on the band in this starting position.
Curl the bands toward your ears and hold the contracted position for two seconds.

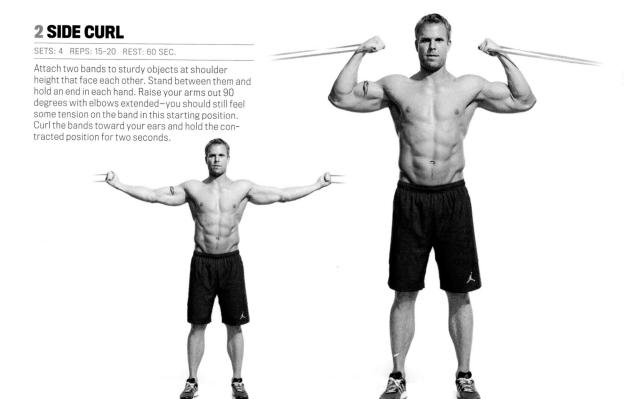

3 REVERSE CURL

SETS: 4   REPS: 15-20 (EACH SIDE)
REST: 60 SEC.

Attach a band to a sturdy object
in front of you and stand facing it.
Hold the band in both hands and
walk backward, adding tension to
the band. Curl the band quickly—
your forearm should end up at 90
degrees or greater to the floor.
Hold the contracted position
for two seconds.

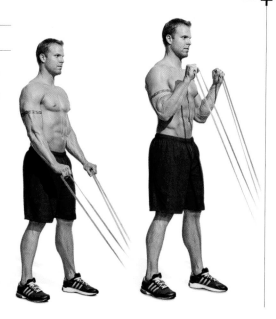

4 HIGH-SPEED CURL

SETS: SEE BELOW   REPS: 50 TOTAL
REST: 60 SEC.

Repeat the first exercise, but use
a higher-tension band, or use
a wider stance to increase the
resistance on the band you have.
Perform only 50 reps this time.

14

TRICEPS

Many guys unfairly focus on their biceps, thinking that the key to bigger arms lies in doing more curls. The truth is that the triceps make up most of the upper arm (two-thirds, in fact), and while they're not as much fun to practice posing in the mirror as their neighbors to the north, they account for more impressive pipes when fully developed.

Bigger, stronger triceps also play a key role in bench pressing and assist on back exercises, so if you want to get your arm-training priorities straight, start with this chapter.

THE BEST
FULL-GYM TRICEPS WORKOUT

WORKOUT #31   BY JIM SMITH, C.S.C.S.

Because the triceps are bigger muscles than the biceps, they can take more of a pounding and respond well to both heavy weight and high reps. Tack on this routine to the end of an upper-body workout to develop triceps size and strength.

HOW IT WORKS The close-grip bench press is one of the all-time great triceps builders because it lets you load heavy weights that recruit all available muscle fibers. Afterward, you'll lighten up on the remaining exercises and go for a big pump, getting as many reps as you can per set and limiting your rest periods. Triceps extensions done on a decline put a stretch on your tri's that forces them to work harder than the conventional version, and band pushdowns allow you to pump out reps fast without perfect form or elbow strain.

DIRECTIONS Perform the exercises as straight sets at the end of an upper-body workout once per week.

1 CLOSE-GRIP BENCH PRESS

SETS: 4 REPS: 8, 8, 8, AS MANY AS POSSIBLE REST: 60 SEC.

Grasp the bar with your index fingers on the inside edge of the knurling (the rough part of the bar). Arch your back so there's space between your lower back and the bench. Pull the bar off the rack and lower it to your sternum, tucking your elbows about 45 degrees to your sides. When the bar touches your body, drive your feet hard into the floor and press the bar back up. On your last set, use half the weight and perform as many reps as possible.

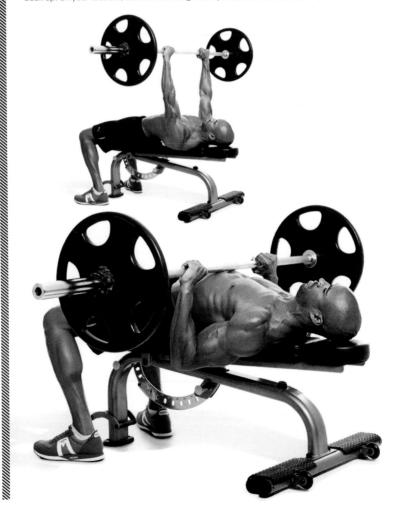

2 DECLINE TRICEPS EXTENSION

SETS: 4   REPS: AS MANY AS POSSIBLE   REST: 15 SEC.

Set an adjustable bench to a slight decline (around 30 degrees) and lie on it with a dumbbell in each hand. Hold the weights over your chest, palms facing each other. Bend your elbows and lower the weights to the sides of your head. Choose a weight you can do 12 reps with on the first set, and use it for every set.

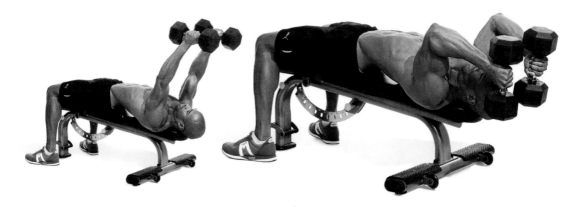

3 BAND PUSHDOWN

SETS: AS MANY AS NEEDED
REPS: 100 TOTAL   REST: AS NEEDED

Attach an elastic exercise band (we like the EFS Pro Light bands from *elitefts.com*) to a sturdy overhead object and grasp each side of the loop. Keeping your elbows tight against your sides, extend your arms downward. You can perform a pushdown on a cable machine instead if you prefer.

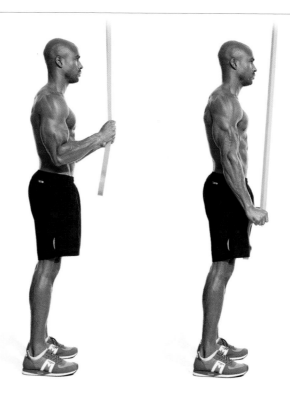

THE BEST BARBELL-ONLY TRICEPS WORKOUT

WORKOUT #32   BY C.J. MURPHY, M.F.S.

When it comes to planning a triceps workout, most people immediately think of cables. While cables certainly lend themselves to productive triceps training, they're far from your only option. In fact, with only a barbell at your disposal, you can blast your triceps while secondarily hitting other upper-body muscle groups, like chest and back.

HOW IT WORKS The pullover is generally used as a back exercise because bringing your arms from behind your head to over your face mainly calls on the lats. But the triceps get involved too—particularly the long head, which runs down the inner side of your arm—assisting the movement. If you think about your triceps while you perform your sets, and actively flex them at the end of each rep, you'll feel them get tired and sore. It's not exactly "The Force," but it does help you get more out of your exercises and the limited equipment you have.

DIRECTIONS Complete all the prescribed sets for one exercise before moving on to the next. If you have an EZ-curl bar instead of or in addition to a straight barbell as shown, feel free to use it as a substitute. It can relieve discomfort of the elbows and wrists. You may also perform the lying triceps extension and pullover on a bench or similarly elevated surface in order to put more of a stretch on the triceps.

1 CLOSE-GRIP FLOOR PRESS

SETS: 5   REPS: 12   REST: 60 SEC.

Lie on the floor and roll the barbell up to your chest or have a partner hand it to you. Grasp the bar at about shoulder width and arch your back so there's space between your lower back and the floor. Lower the bar to your sternum, tucking your elbows about 45 degrees to your sides. When your triceps touch the floor (not your elbows), press the bar back up.

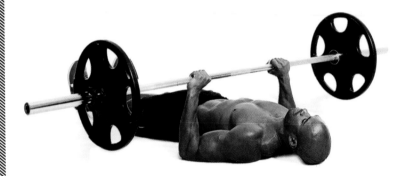

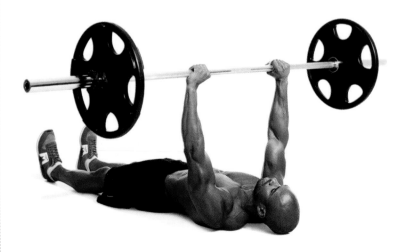

2 LYING TRICEPS EXTENSION

SETS: 4   REPS: 20   REST: 60 SEC.

Press the bar over your chest and then let your upper arms drift back to about a 45-degree angle. Bend your elbows to lower the bar behind your head, and then extend them to return to the starting position. Keep your elbows in line with your wrists throughout.

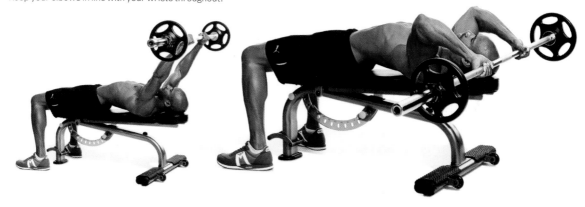

3 PULLOVER

SETS: 3   REPS: 12-15   REST: 60 SEC.

Hold the bar overhead with an overhand, shoulder-width grip and lie back on the floor. Press the bar over your head and then reach back over your head, bending your elbows only slightly. Continue until you feel a stretch in your lats, and then pull the bar back over your chest, flexing your triceps as you go. Focus your mind on your triceps and you'll feel them engage more throughout the exercise.

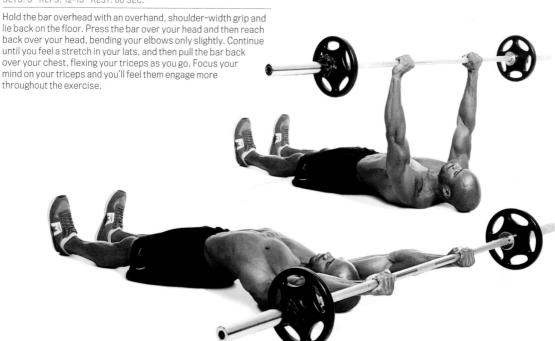

THE BEST DUMBBELL-ONLY TRICEPS WORKOUT

WORKOUT #33   BY MICHAEL SCHLETTER, C.P.T.

The triceps is made up of three parts, hence the "tri"–apologies if this insults your intelligence. The inner side of the muscle that runs down your arm closest to your body is known as the long head, and the lateral and medial heads appear on the outer portion of the arm. These are the parts of the muscle that are most visible when you're wearing a T-shirt and the two you'll want to focus on for next summer with this workout.

HOW IT WORKS Our program targets the lateral and medial heads with exercises you're probably unfamiliar with. This is all the better to encourage growth. The Tate press can also improve your lockout on bench presses, while the underhand kickback provides some extra grip and forearm training.

DIRECTIONS Perform the exercise pairs (marked "A" and "B") as supersets. So you'll do a set of A and then a set of B before resting. Repeat for all the prescribed sets. Exercise 3 is done with conventional straight sets.

1A NEUTRAL-GRIP PRESS

SETS: 4 REPS; 8-12 REST: 0 SEC.

Hold a dumbbell in each hand and lie back on a bench (if available) or a low box or other surface that raises your body slightly above the floor. Hold the dumbbells at shoulder level with palms facing each other. Press them over your chest.

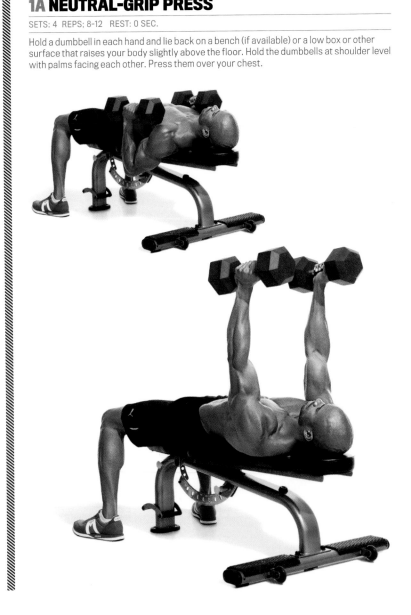

1B LYING TRICEPS EXTENSION

SETS: 4   REPS: 8-12   REST: 120 SEC.

From the end position of your last rep of the neutral-grip press, allow your arms to drift
back until the weights are over your face. Keeping your upper arms at that angle, bend
your elbows and lower the weights behind your head. Extend your elbows, keeping the
same angle with your upper arms.

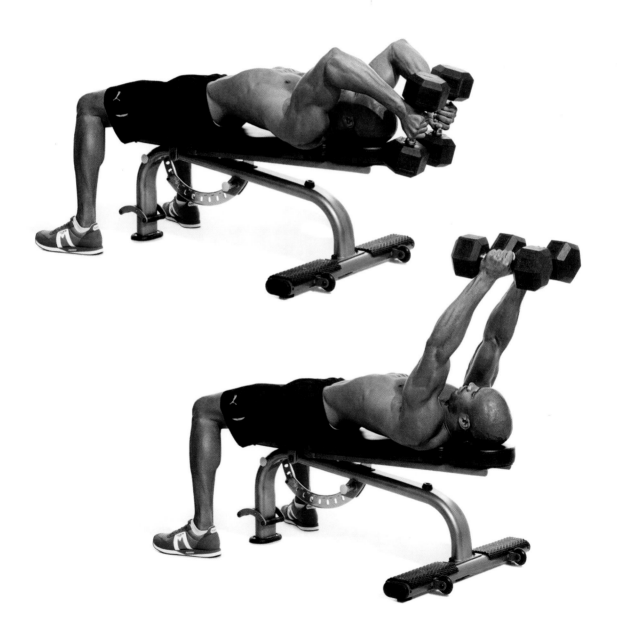

2A TATE PRESS

SETS: 4 REPS: 8-12 REST: 0 SEC.

Lie back on a bench or surface with dumbbells in each hand,
arms extended over your chest and palms facing your feet. Point
your elbows outward and bend them to lower the weights almost
to your chest, so they make L shapes. Extend your elbows.

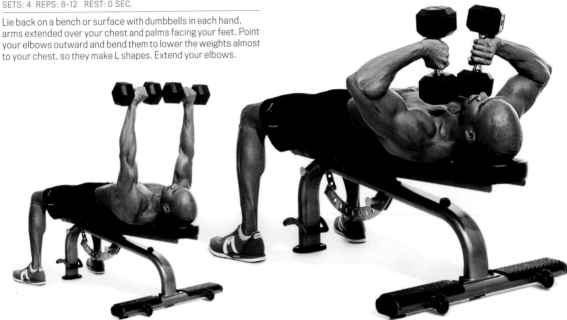

2B UNDERHAND KICKBACK

SETS: 4 REPS: 8-12 REST: 120 SEC.

Stand holding a dumbbell in each
hand and bend your hips back,
lowering your torso until it's almost
parallel to the floor. Turn your palms
to face in front of you and, keeping
your upper arms against your sides,
extend your elbows until your arms
are parallel to your torso.

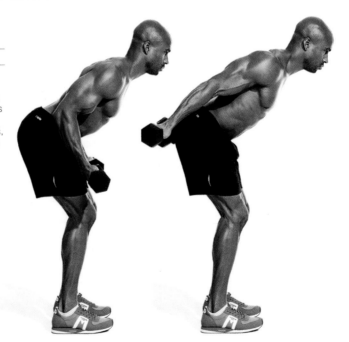

3 ONE-ARM OVERHEAD EXTENSION

SETS: 4   REPS: 8-12 (EACH SIDE)   REST: 120 SEC.

Hold one dumbbell and raise your arm behind your head with your elbow bent. Extend your elbow to point your arm straight overhead.

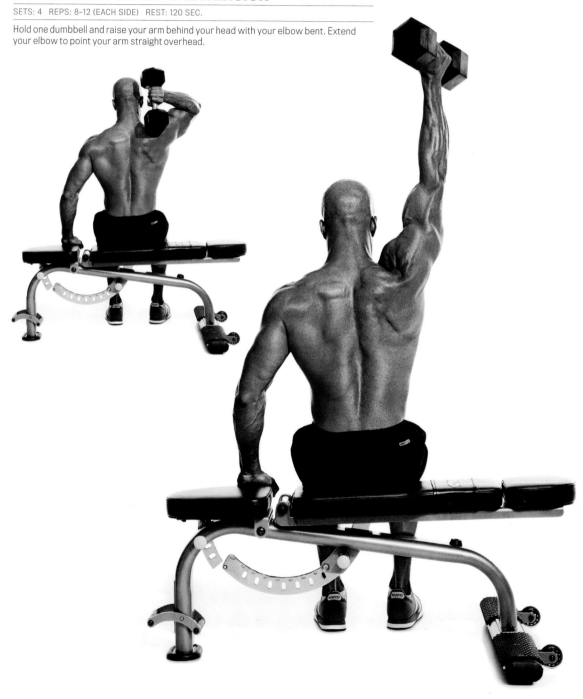

THE BEST BAND-ONLY TRICEPS WORKOUT

WORKOUT #34   BY JIM SMITH, C.S.C.S.

Bands are inexpensive, lightweight, versatile, and ideal for training triceps. We've made this routine customizable to whatever bands you have available. Regardless of the tension or the design, you'll get adequate work to make your triceps grow.

HOW IT WORKS When trainers write workouts for clients they haven't met (in this case, you), they often prescribe doing reps for a certain amount of time. So whether an exercise is easy or hard for you, you'll be able to get something out of it (i.e., you'll do more reps if it's easy and fewer if it's hard). The band exercises we're giving you work that way, and body-weight training makes up the rest.

DIRECTIONS Perform the exercise pairs (marked "A" and "B") as supersets. So you'll do a set of A and then a set of B before resting. Repeat for all the prescribed sets.

1A DIP

SETS: 4   REPS: 10   REST: 0 SEC.

Use dip bars if available, or place your palms on a bench or chair and extend your legs in front of you. Lower your body until your upper arms are parallel to the floor, but no lower. Extend your elbows to come up.

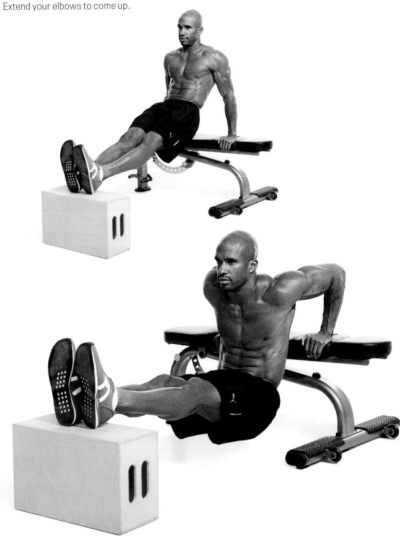

1B TRICEPS EXTENSION

SETS: 4 REPS/TIME: 30 SEC.
REST: 90 SEC.

Attach the band to a sturdy overhead
object and grasp the free end (or
handles) with both hands. Tuck
your elbows to your sides and
extend your elbows to lockout.

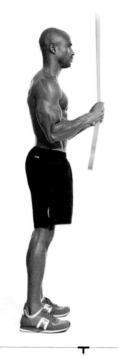
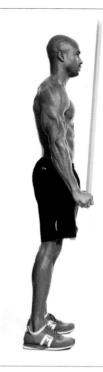

2A CLOSE-GRIP PUSHUP

SETS: 4 REPS: 20 REST: 0 SEC.

Get into pushup position with your hands inside shoulder width.
Keeping your abs braced, lower your body until your chest is
just above the floor and then push up. For an advanced workout, use the band for resistance by wrapping it around your
back and holding an end in each hand.

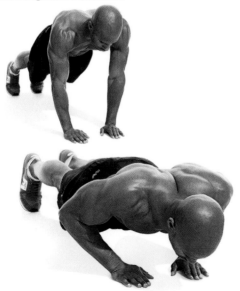

2B DOUBLE-BAND TRICEPS EXTENSION

SETS: 4 REPS/TIME: 30 SEC.   REST: 90 SEC.

Set up as you did for the triceps extensions, but attach a second
band to the loop of the first one. Grab the ends of the second
band and perform triceps extensions with a slight bend in
your hips.

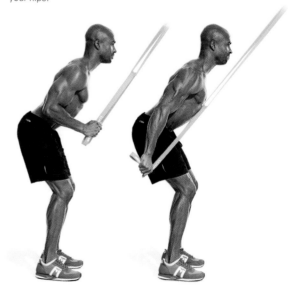

THE BEST BODY-WEIGHT TRICEPS WORKOUT

WORKOUT #35   BY C.J. MURPHY, M.F.S.

We usually don't rec-ommend leaving your fitness to chance, but a deck of cards can liven up your rou-tine and provide a surprisingly well-tailored workout. Take a gamble on this approach and you'll see your triceps grow.

HOW IT WORKS All you need is your own body weight and a deck of cards. You'll let the deck determine the number of reps you perform for the diamond pushup—the best pushup vari-ation for targeting the triceps. It may seem random, but you'll end up getting plenty of push-ups done, and when you don't have weights to apply a more strenuous load to your muscles, giving them a high volume of work is the only way to induce enough muscle damage to result in growth. The remaining two exercises follow the same thinking, as you aim for 100 total reps on a tough triceps exten-sion variant and go for as many as possible on dips.

DIRECTIONS Complete all the prescribed sets for one exercise before moving on to the next.

1 DIAMOND PUSHUP W/CARDS

SETS: 3   REPS: SEE BELOW   REST: SEE BELOW

Place a deck of cards on the floor and randomly select some to make three stacks of 10 each. Place the cards facedown. The numbers on the cards will be the number of reps you'll perform—face cards count as 10, and aces may be wild but no less than 10.

Flip a card in one pile and perform the number of reps it calls for. Rest 20 seconds and then flip another card. Continue until you've completed that stack and then rest two minutes. Repeat the process with the remaining two stacks.

To perform the diamond pushup, get into pushup position with your hands close together so that your index fingers and thumbs touch and form a diamond shape. Keeping your abs braced and torso in line with your hips, lower your body until your chest nearly touches the floor.

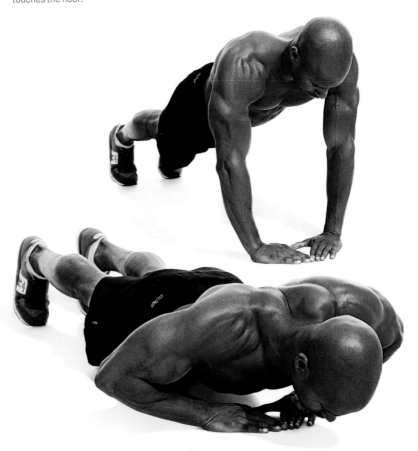

2 TRICEPS EXTENSION

SETS: AS MANY AS NEEDED
REPS: 100 TOTAL   REST: 60 SEC.

Use an elevated surface that's about waist height and can support your weight, such as a windowsill. Place your hands on it at shoulder width and let it support your weight, with your torso and hips in line and abs braced. Bend your elbows to lower your head beneath the object until you feel a stretch on your triceps. Now extend your elbows to come back up. Perform 100 total reps, taking as many sets as needed to hit that number.

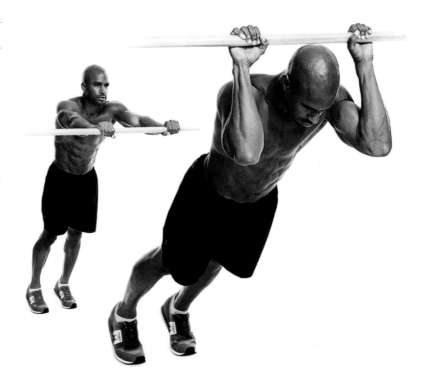

3 HALF DIP

SETS: 5   REPS: AS MANY AS POSSIBLE   REST: 60 SEC.

Place your palms on a bench or chair and extend your legs in front of you. Lower your body halfway to the floor and then extend your elbows to come up. Try to explode upward on each rep.

15 FOREARMS

Direct forearm training is usually performed at the end of an upper-body or arm workout, but there's no reason you can't give them their own day if you want. In addition to the workouts we've provide here, there are some other steps you can take to bolster your forearm gains. Avoid using wrist straps on your back exercises, especially the deadlift. The harder you can squeeze your hands around a bar—and the heavier that bar is—the more forearm muscle you'll activate.

THE BEST FULL-GYM FOREARM WORKOUT

WORKOUT #36   BY MARTIN ROONEY

A gym towel can be used for more than soaking up sweat and protecting your modesty in the locker room. When used as a handle, it's a cheap, portable, and highly effective tool for beefing up your forearms.

HOW IT WORKS The forearms are best activated by exercises that have you pulling and squeezing. Using a towel as an attachment for cable rows and pullups intensifies muscle recruitment. Although this workout targets your forearms, you can't help but strengthen your back and biceps doing these exercises as well. After a few weeks, you'll probably notice that conventional barbells, dumbbells, and cable attachments feel thin as pencils.

DIRECTIONS Perform the workout one day per week, spaced at least a day between any other back or biceps training. Hold the top (contracted) position in each rep for one second. Complete all sets for one exercise before going on to the next.

1 TOWEL CABLE ROW

SETS: 3 REPS: 8 REST: 60 SEC.

Hook a towel to a cable pulley and stand in front of it. Set up to do a row, holding an end of the towel in each hand. Squeeze your shoulder blades together and row the towel to your rib cage.

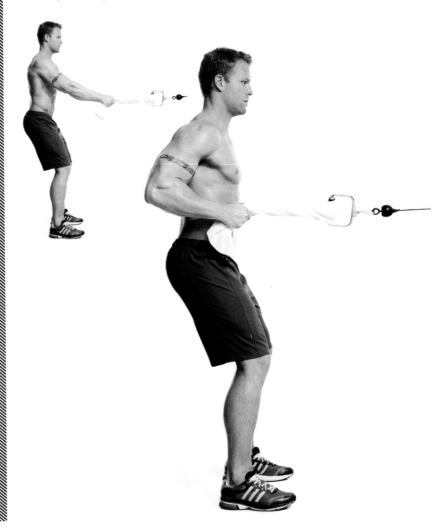

2 TOWEL ROW TO CHEST

SETS: 5 REPS: 7 REST: 60 SEC.

Loop a towel around the bar of a lat-pulldown machine and hold an end of the towel in each hand. Your arms should be extended and at eye level. Brace one foot on the seat of the machine and pull the bar to your chest as in a normal row.

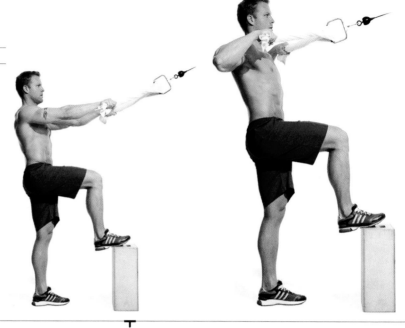

3 TOWEL PULLUP

SETS: 4 REPS: 5 REST: 90 SEC.

Hang a towel over a pullup bar and grasp an end in each hand. Hang from the towel and then pull yourself up until your chin is above your hands. If that's too difficult, simply hang from the towel for as long as you can.

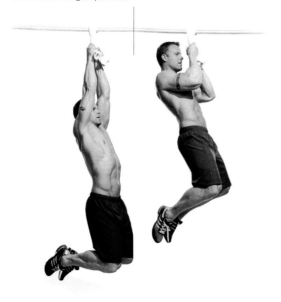

4 TOWEL KETTLEBELL CURL

SETS: 3 REPS: 6 (EACH SIDE) REST: 90 SEC.

Run the towel through the handle of a kettlebell, or wrap two towels around a pair of dumbbells as shown, and fold it in half. Hold both ends in one hand (for kettlebell), or both ends in each hand (dumbbells) and curl, keeping your upper arm stationary.

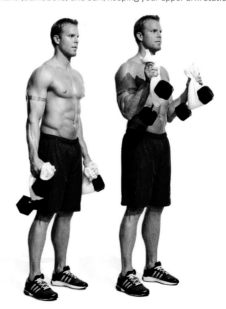

THE BEST DUMBBELL-ONLY FOREARM WORKOUT

WORKOUT #37   BY JIM SMITH, C.S.C.S.

There are a number of rules you have to follow when training muscles like the pecs, biceps, and thighs: Use a full range of motion, hold at the top, use strict form, etc. Thankfully, forearms are a bit simpler–just squeeze.

HOW IT WORKS Gripping heavy weights and holding on is pretty much all it takes to make your forearms blow up. Just picture a construction worker, strongman competitor, or heavy deadlifter–they all sport impressive forearms even if they don't spend much or any time training them directly.

That's the main goal with this workout. Handle as heavy weights as possible for as long as you can before letting them drop (and hopefully not on your toes). The farmer's walk may sound easy but it's one of the most exhausting exercises you can perform, and not just for the forearms, but every part of you. You'll also focus on lowering various curls slowly, controlling the negative portion of the rep. This induces the greatest muscle damage and soreness, and results in forearms like bowling pins.

DIRECTIONS Perform exercises 3A and 3B as supersets. So you'll do a set of A and then a set of B before resting. Repeat for all the prescribed sets. Perform the remaining exercises as straight sets, completing all sets for one move before going on to the next.

1 FARMER'S WALK

SETS: 3   REPS: WALK 40-50 YARDS
REST: 120 SEC.

Pick up the heaviest dumbbells you can handle and walk with your chest out, standing tall with arms at your sides. Go 40-50 yards–you can walk in a figure-eight pattern if you don't have the space. At the end of the distance, stop and continue to hold the weights for as long as possible.

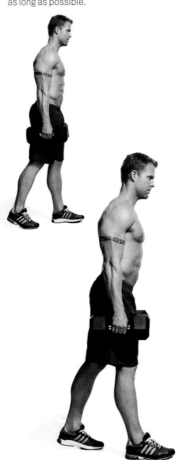

2 HAMMER CHEAT CURL

SETS: 3   REPS: 8   REST: 60 SEC.

Grasp a dumbbell in each hand and cheat the weights, as if doing a clean, to the top position of a curl. Use momentum from your hips to get the weights up. Slowly lower the weights back down for five counts.

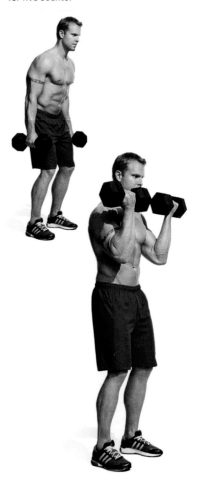

3A WRIST CURL

SETS: 3   REPS: 15   REST: 0 SEC.

Hold a dumbbell in each hand and sit on a bench, box, or chair. Rest your forearms on your thighs and allow your wrists to bend back over your knees so the weights hang down. Curl the dumbbells up by just flexing your wrists.

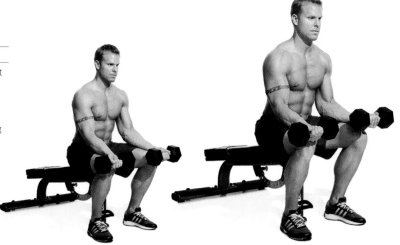

3B REVERSE WRIST CURL

SETS: 3   REPS: 15   REST: 90 SEC.

Perform the opposite motion of the wrist curl. Palms face down and extend your wrists to raise the back of your hands closer to your forearms.

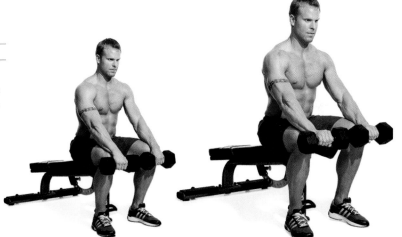

4 GRIP CRUSH

SETS: 3   REPS: AS MANY AS POSSIBLE
REST: 120 SEC.

Sit on a bench, box, or chair with a dumbbell in your left. Extend your arm toward the floor and brace the back of it against the inside of your left thigh. Allow your hand to open and the dumbbell to roll to your fingertips. Now close your hand and perform a wrist curl, squeezing the weight as hard as possible. Choose a weight you could perform 8-12 normal biceps curls with.

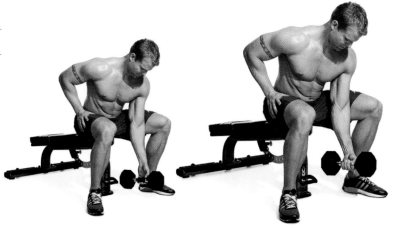

THE BEST BARBELL-ONLY FOREARM WORKOUT

WORKOUT #38   BY C.J. MURPHY, M.F.S.

If you're a minimalist, then you've got to love when you can do your normal workout and get a whole new muscle-building stimulus out of it with almost no extra effort. In fact, one way to get great forearms is to do the same curling exercises you typically would but with a towel around the bar to increase the recruitment of forearm muscles. This workout makes minor tweaks to a basic arm routine to render it twice as effective.

HOW IT WORKS Using a towel makes curls, which normally hit just the biceps, incorporate more of the forearm. To take it a step further, we're prescribing reverse curls later in the workout to target the brachioradialis (the long forearm muscle that points to your thumb) and brachialis (a cylinder of muscle between your biceps and triceps), but your biceps will still get hit hard at the same time. You don't mind that, do you?

DIRECTIONS Complete all the prescribed sets for one exercise before moving on to the next.

1 TOWEL CURL

SETS: 3   REPS: 12-15, 10-12, 6-8   REST: 60 SEC.

Loop a thick towel around the bar so that it doesn't let your hands close all the way when you grasp it. Hold the bar with an overhand, shoulder-width grip, in front of your thighs. Without allowing your upper arms to move forward, curl the bar. Add weight each set so you must reduce your reps.

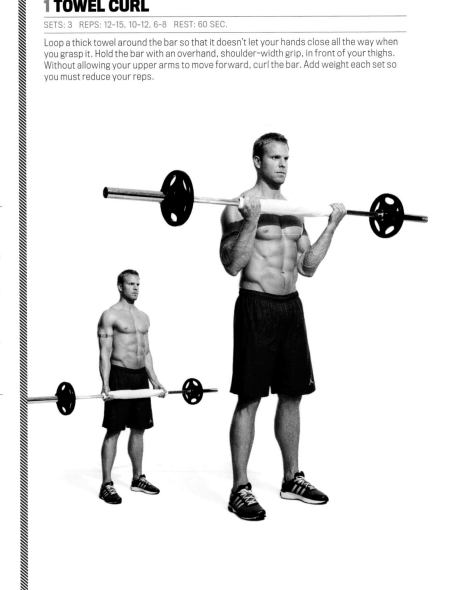

2 REVERSE CURL

SETS: 3   REPS: 12   REST: 60 SEC.

Grasp the bar overhand at whatever width is comfortable. Keeping your upper arms against your sides, curl the bar.

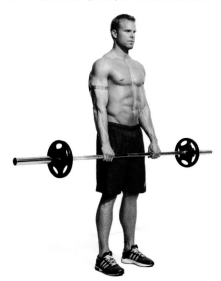

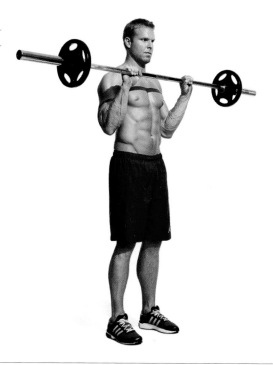

3 REVERSE CURL 21

SETS: 2   REPS: 7 (EACH POSITION)   REST: 60 SEC.

Curl the bar halfway up and hold for one second. Lower it back and repeat for six more reps. Then curl the bar to the mid point and, beginning there, curl it all the way up for seven reps, using the mid point as the "bottom" of each rep. Finally, perform seven full-range reps.

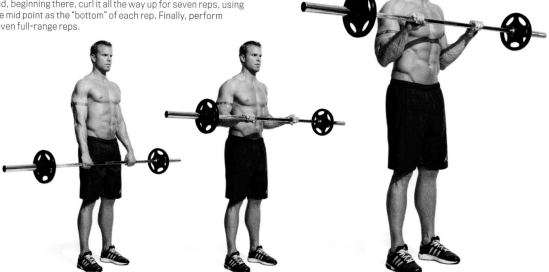

16

CHEST

The pecs are worked mainly with press and flye movements (and a few other interesting ways you're about to discover for the first time). Despite the simplicity of how these muscles work, they can be trained with a variety of implements, each of which offers its own special pec-building properties. Machines, barbells, dumbbells, suspension trainers, medicine balls, bands, and body weight all provide strategies to make your shirts tight enough to test the integrity of their buttons.

THE BEST FULL-GYM CHEST WORKOUT [option A]

WORKOUT #39   BY HANY RAMBOD

Bodybuilders of the '70s liked to stretch and flex the muscles they were training between sets, believing it enhanced growth. What they stumbled upon has been refined into a formal muscle-building protocol by Hany Rambod, trainer to many of today's top champions including Mr. Olympia winners Phil Heath and Jay Cutler. Here, we use his FST-7 method to pack new meat on your pecs.

HOW IT WORKS After pounding the pectorals with some conventional chest exercises, we finish them off with FST-7, which stands for "Fascial Stretch Training" done for seven sets. Fascial refers to the fascia, the web-like connective tissue that envelopes each muscle. Picture that thin layer that covers a skinless chicken breast—that's the same stuff. By stretching the fascia, you create more room for the muscles to grow. By flexing, you'll drive more nutrient-filled blood into the muscles to enhance gains.

DIRECTIONS Every set should be taken to near failure. For the cable crossover, alternate stretching and then flexing your pecs between sets. So you'll complete a set and then stretch for 30 seconds, then do another set and flex for 30 seconds. After the stretch/flex, you can rest up to 45 seconds.
For the stretch, rest your forearms against a doorframe, or use the beams of a power rack, and lean forward. To flex, tense your pecs isometrically.

1 SMITH MACHINE INCLINE PRESS

SETS: 4   REPS: 10-12   REST: 60-90 SEC.

Set an adjustable bench to a 30- to 45-degree incline, and roll it into the center of a Smith machine rack. Grasp the bar with an overhand, shoulder-width grip. Unrack the bar, lower it to the upper part of your chest, and press straight up.

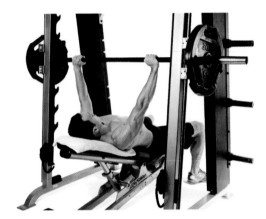

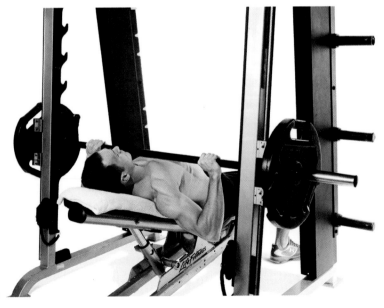

2 DUMBBELL BENCH PRESS

SETS: 3   REPS: 10-12   REST: 60-90 SEC.

Lie back on a flat bench with a dumbbell in each hand. Hold the weights at shoulder level and then press the weights straight over your chest.

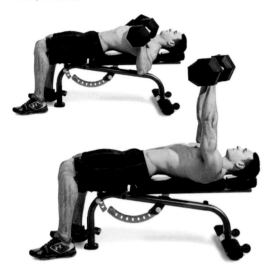

3 INCLINE DUMBBELL FLYE

SETS: 3   REPS: 10-12   REST: 60-90 SEC.

Set an adjustable bench to a 30- to 45-degree angle and lie back on it with a dumbbell in each hand. Turn your wrists so your palms face each other. Press the weights straight over your chest and then, keeping a slight bend in your elbows, spread your arms open as if you were going for a big bear hug. Lower your arms until you feel a stretch in your pecs and then bring the weights back together over your chest.

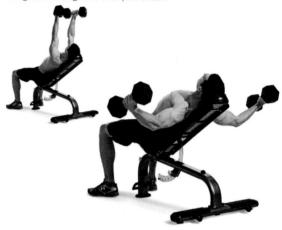

4 BENCH PRESS

SETS: 3   REPS: 10-12   REST: 60-90 SEC.

Grasp the bar just outside shoulder width and arch your back so there's space between your lower back and the bench. Pull the bar out of the rack and lower it to your sternum, tucking your elbows about 45 degrees to your sides. When the bar touches your body, drive your feet hard into the floor and press the bar back up.

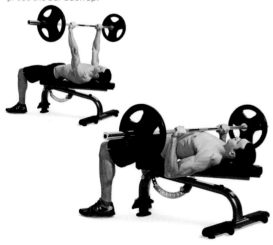

5 CABLE CROSSOVER

SETS: 7   REPS: 10   REST: 30-45 SECONDS

Stand between two facing cable stations with both pulleys set midway between the top and bottom of the station. Attach a D-handle to each pulley and hold one in each hand. Keep your elbows slightly bent and step forward so there's tension on the cables. Flex your pecs as you bring your hands together out in front of your chest. Alternate stretching and flexing after each set.

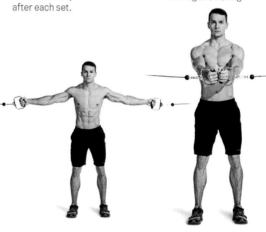

THE BEST FULL-GYM CHEST WORKOUT [option B]

WORKOUT #40   BY HANY RAMBOD

■ If you've been working out for a while, this routine will probably remind you of some of the chest sessions you did in the early days. It's good, old-fashioned hard work and provides a lot of isolation of the pecs. If you've gotten more scientific with your training since and noticed fewer gains, this simple and direct approach may be what you need to get growing again.

HOW IT WORKS When a muscle contracts, the whole thing contracts. So when you hear trainers talking about exercises for the "upper" pecs and "inner" pecs, this isn't entirely accurate. However, while the whole pectoralis major muscle is involved in any kind of press, dip, or flye motion, different parts of it are indeed emphasized depending on the angle of resistance. So while an incline dumbbell press will work the whole chest, it's making the fibers that attach to your clavicle work harder than the ones that attach to your ribs.

We've given you exercises that work every part of the chest and with varying degrees of isolation. If you don't normally feel your pecs working on barbell presses, you'll love what dumbbell and machine work does for you.

DIRECTIONS Stop each set a rep or two short of failure.

Feel free to combine the workout with Option A, shown previously. The two routines fit well together but should be spaced three days apart.

1 INCLINE DUMBBELL PRESS

SETS: 4   REPS: 8   REST: 60-90 SEC.

Set an adjustable bench to a 30- to 45-degree angle and lie back on it with a dumbbell in each hand at shoulder level. Press the weights over your chest.

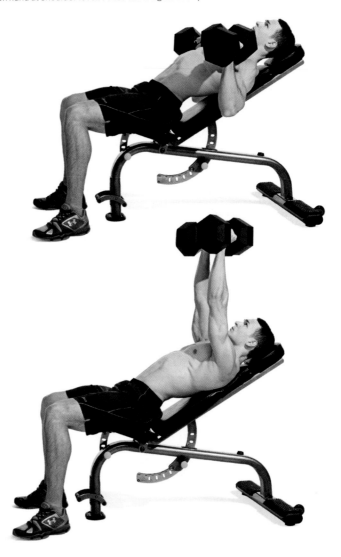

2 HAMMER STRENGTH CHEST PRESS

SETS: 4   REPS: 8   REST: 60-90 SEC.

Use a Hammer Strength flat-press machine if you can and adjust the seat so that both of your feet are flat on the floor. Grasp the handles and press to a full lockout.

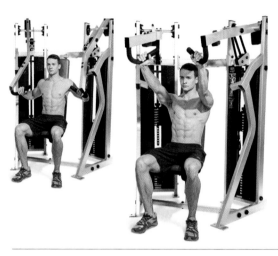

3 DUMBBELL FLYE

SETS: 3   REPS: 8   REST: 60-90 SEC.

Lie back on a flat bench with a dumbbell in each hand. Keep a slight bend in your elbows and spread your arms wide, lowering the weights until they're even with your chest. Flex your pecs and lift the weights back to the starting position.

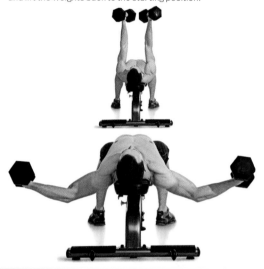

4 LOW-CABLE CROSSOVER

SETS: 3   REPS: 8   REST: 60-90 SEC.

Stand between two facing cable stations and attach a D-handle to the low pulleys on each. With a handle in each hand and elbows slightly bent, raise your arms from waist height to out in front of your chest, flexing your pecs as you bring them together.

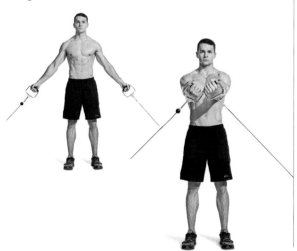

5 DIP

SETS: 4   REPS: 8   REST: 60-90 SEC.

Suspend yourself over the bars of a dip station and lower your body until your upper arms are parallel to the floor. If eight reps is too easy, add weight using a weighted belt or by holding a dumbbell between your feet.

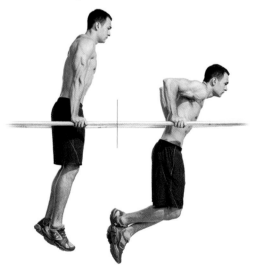

THE BEST BARBELL-ONLY CHEST WORKOUT

WORKOUT #41   BY JASON FERRUGGIA

There are three training methods that have proven effective for building muscle: using heavy weights, doing lots of reps, and lifting explosively. The first two are familiar to you, but you probably haven't thought much about the third–known as speed work. Combine all three and your chest will have to grow.

HOW IT WORKS We want you to perform the classic bench press on a slight incline. Not only is it safer for your shoulders, but it also brings the pecs more strongly into the movement. The speed bench press is done light, but that doesn't mean easy. Light weights travel faster, and your goal should be to make every rep move at warp speed. Explosive reps activate the most powerful muscle fibers and also help you overcome sticking points in your bench press.

DIRECTIONS Complete all sets for one exercise before moving on to the next.

1 LOW-INCLINE PRESS

SETS: 3   REPS: 6-8   REST: 90 SEC.

Set an adjustable bench to an incline of no more than 30 degrees, or rest a flat bench on a weight plate or mat to tilt it slightly. Grasp the bar just outside shoulder width and arch your back so there's space between your lower back and the bench. Pull the bar out of the rack and lower it to your sternum, tucking your elbows about 45 degrees to your sides. When the bar touches your body, drive your feet hard into the floor and press the bar back up.

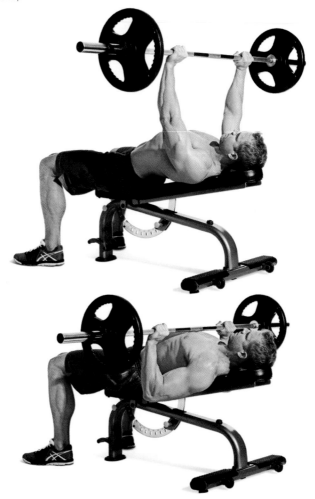

2 SPEED BENCH PRESS

SETS: 3   REPS: 5   REST: 60 SEC.

Bench press as described at left, but do so on a totally flat
bench. Use 60% of your max. So if you think you can bench-
press 250 pounds one time, perform your sets with 150,
exploding each rep off your chest as fast as you can.

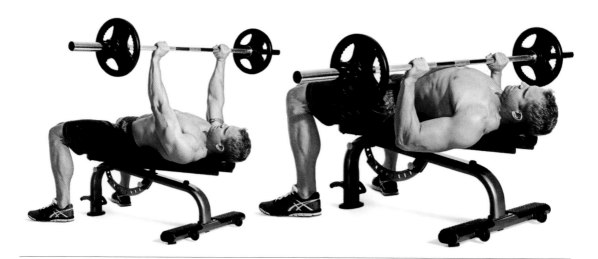

3 LANDMINE PRESS

SETS: 3   REPS: 8, 10, 15 (EACH SIDE)   REST: 60 SEC.

Wedge the end of the barbell into a corner of the room (to avoid
damage to the walls, you may have to wrap a towel around it).
Load the opposite end with weight and grasp it toward the end
of the sleeve with your left hand. Stagger your stance so your
right leg is in front. Press the bar straight overhead.

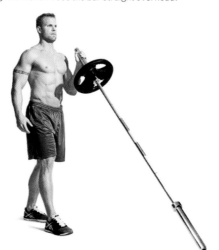

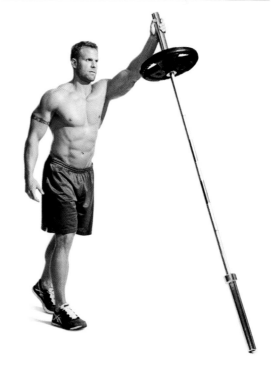

THE BEST DUMBBELL-ONLY CHEST WORKOUT

WORKOUT #42   BY C.J. MURPHY, M.F.S.

Chest training is always done with some kind of bench. You need something to brace your back while you press or flye, and hold you in position while your pecs get a stretch. But what if you don't have a bench handy, which is a definite possibility in a small hotel gym, or your garage, where all you've invested in so far is some selectorized dumbbells? Here's how to get a chest workout so effective you won't even miss the bench.

HOW IT WORKS Lacking something to stabilize your upper body just means you'll have to do it yourself, which is fine—the exercises will be harder, but they'll activate more stabilizer muscles in the chest, back, shoulders, and core. Really, your training won't seem that different. You can still press like you're benching, but you'll do it on the floor. You can still do flyes, but you'll do them from pushup position (you'll see). The plate pressout, however, will likely be a brand-new challenge for you. You'll be amazed how strong a contraction you can get in your pecs without heavy weights or a bench to lie on.

DIRECTIONS Complete all sets for one exercise before moving on to the next.

1 FLOOR PRESS

SETS: 4   REPS: 8   REST: 60 SEC.

Lie on the floor with a dumbbell in each hand. Your palms should face each other and your triceps should be resting on the floor, but not your elbows. Explosively press the dumbbells up. Lower them until only your triceps touch the floor. Pause for a moment and then begin the next rep. Increase the weight gradually each set.

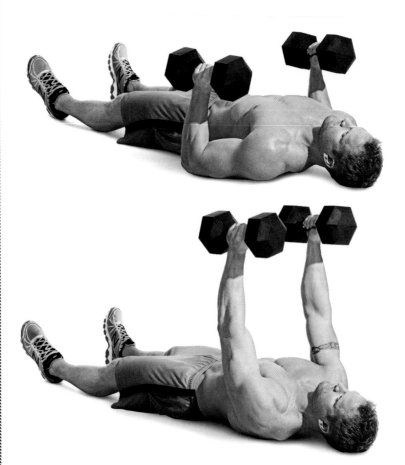

2 PRONE FLYE

SETS: 4   REPS: AS MANY AS POSSIBLE   REST: 60 SEC.

Hold a dumbbell in each hand and get into pushup position on the floor with palms facing each other. Spread your arms apart as in a normal dumbbell flye and lower your body until you feel a stretch in your chest, then squeeze the dumbbells and bring your hands back to pushup position. Keep your abs and glutes braced and your back flat throughout. If you're using plate-loaded dumbbells, you may be able to roll the weight plates on the floor during the flye. Otherwise, you can place a towel under each dumbbell to facilitate sliding. If this is too difficult, perform the exercise on your knees.

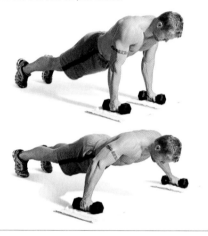

3 PULLOVER

SETS: 3   REPS: 12-15   REST: 60 SEC.

Lie on your back on the floor and hold one dumbbell overhead with both hands. Press the weight over your chest and then reach back over your head, bending your elbows only slightly. Continue until you feel a stretch in your lats, and then pull the dumbbell back over your chest. Take a deep breath every time you lower the dumbbell behind you.

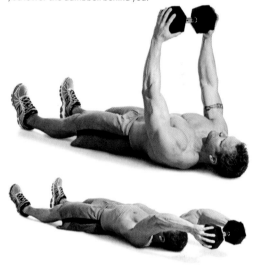

4 PLATE PRESSOUT

SETS: 3   REPS: 12-20   REST: 60 SEC.

Hold a pair of light weight plates together, smooth side out, between your palms right in front of your chest. You should look like you're praying. Squeeze the plates together, focusing on your chest, and press them out in front of you until your arms are extended. Flare your lats and pull the weights back to your chest. Complete your reps and then, on the second set, press the weights downward from your chest at a 45-degree angle. On the third set, press them upward at a 45-degree angle.

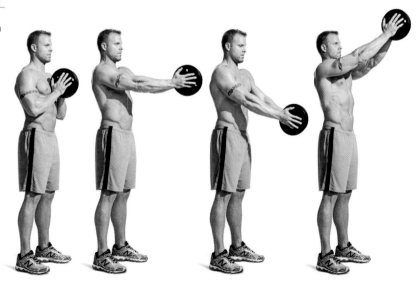

THE BEST SUSPENSION-TRAINER CHEST WORKOUT

WORKOUT #43   BY BEN BRUNO

When a guy wants to get a big chest, he tends to make the classic mistake of training only his chest–or training it twice as often and as hard as any other body part. Even if shirt-popping pecs is all you're interested in, you'll get faster results if you train the rest of the body, too, particularly the upper back and shoulders. The routine at right addresses all three.

HOW IT WORKS The more muscle you add to one side of your body, the more you need to add to the opposite side in order to keep the balance. If you don't, the body will eventually forbid muscle growth to the area that has grown out of whack, because it doesn't want to risk the injury. This is one of the most common and easily preventable ways to plateau.

You'll target your chest very specifically in this routine with moves like the three-way flye, which is borrowed from gymnastics training. The pec activation is like nothing you've tried before, so prepare to be sore. However, to keep your upper back and shoulders growing in conjunction with your pecs, we've thrown in some rows, reverse flyes, external rotations, and face pulls. Think of it as a way to build your chest without breaking it.

DIRECTIONS Perform the exercise pairs (marked "A" and "B") as alternating sets. So you'll do a set of A, rest, then a set of B, rest again, and continue for all the prescribed sets.

1A 3-WAY FLYE

SETS: 3 REPS: 3 REST: 90 SEC.

Attach a suspension trainer to a sturdy overhead object and lengthen the straps to a point at which you would to do pushups. Grasp the handles and get into pushup position with hands under your shoulders. Your entire body should be straight and your core braced. Bring your arms out to your sides as if you were giving someone a bear hug. Lower your body until you feel a stretch in your chest and then bring your arms together again. That's one rep of the flye. Perform three reps.

Now, from the starting position, open your arms but keep your elbows bent so that the move looks like a combination of a pushup and a flye. Press yourself back up. That's one rep of the bent-arm flye. Perform three reps.

From there, return to the starting position and perform pushups on the handles. Perform three reps.

All of the above equals one set.

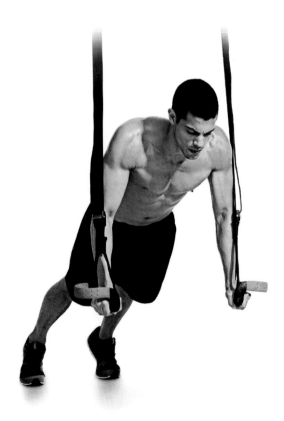

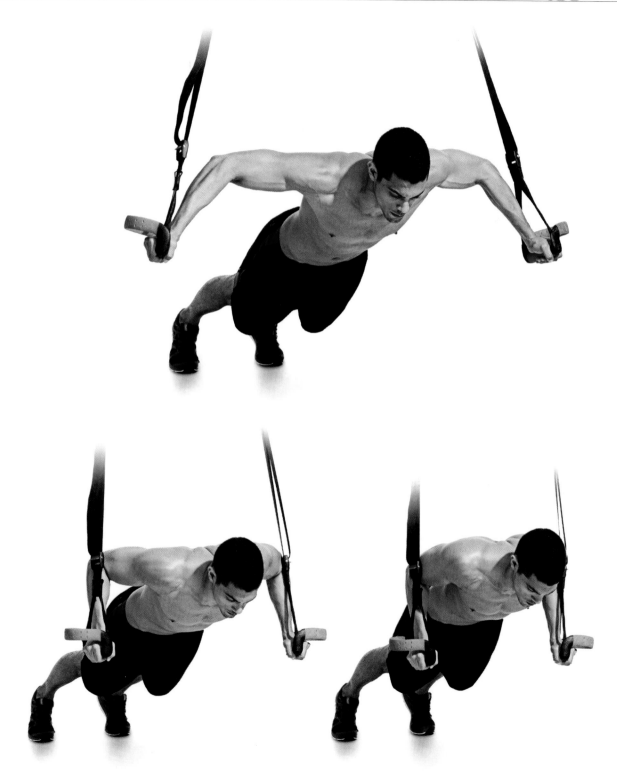

1B INVERTED ROW

SETS: 2   REPS: 12   REST: 90 SEC.

Hold the handles and lean back with arms extended so that your body is supported by the trainer and only your feet are on the floor. Brace your core and hold your body in a straight line. (The lower you set the handles, the harder the exercise; you can elevate your feet on something to make it even harder.) Row your body up until your chest is by your hands and your back is fully contracted. Rotate your wrists as you row your palms up in the end position.

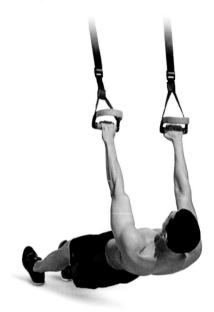

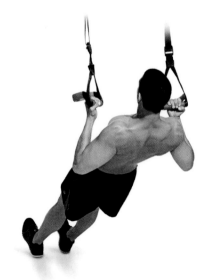

2A PUSHUP

SETS: 3   REPS: 12–15   REST: 90 SEC.

Grasp the handles and get into pushup position with hands under your shoulders. Your entire body should be straight and your core braced. Lower your body until your chest is between the handles.

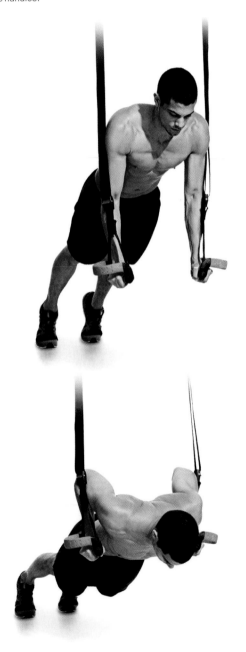

2B 3-WAY FINISHER

SETS: 2 REPS: 5 REST: 120 SEC.

Grasp the handles and lean back away from the trainer's attachment point so that your weight is on your heels and your body is 45–50 degrees to the floor. Allow your arms to extend in front of you. Squeeze your shoulder blades together and draw your arms back until they're 90 degrees out to your sides. (Keep a slight bend in your elbows.) That's one rep of the reverse flye. Perform five reps.

Now, from the start position of the reverse flye, draw your upper arms back with your elbows bent 90 degrees and knuckles facing the ceiling. Your upper body should make a W shape. That's one rep of the external rotation. Perform five reps.

From there, return to the starting position with arms extended and pull your hands to your forehead, twisting your palms to face in front of you as you pull. That's one face pull. Perform five reps.

All of the above equals one set.

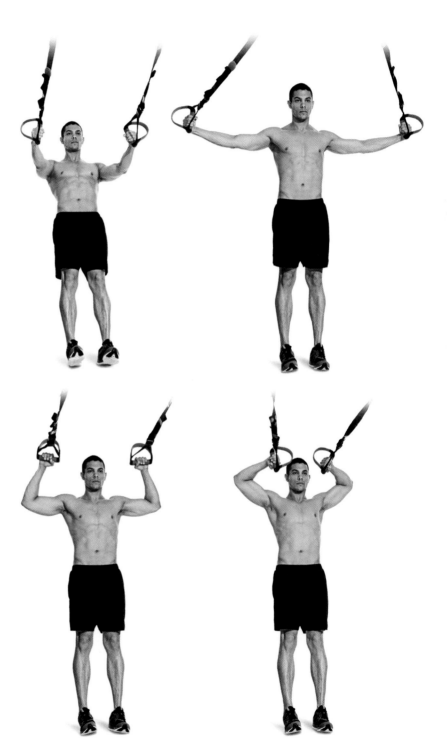

THE BEST
MEDICINE-BALL CHEST WORKOUT

WORKOUT #44   BY NICK TUMMINELLO

This workout takes only 10 minutes and works the triceps hard in addition to the chest. If you don't have a medicine ball, a firm soccer or basketball will work.

HOW IT WORKS A medicine ball is so versatile it doesn't even have to move and it can still help you build muscle. You don't have to throw, catch, or even lift it, but merely use it to balance on. Working to keep it stable will work your own stabilizing muscles in your core, and using it for pushup variations will light up your pecs and triceps.

DIRECTIONS Perform the exercises as a circuit, completing one set of each back to back without rest. Do at least five reps per move and try to add one rep each time you repeat the workout. Complete one to three circuits, resting three to five minutes between each.

1 LOCK-OFF

SETS: 1-3   REPS: 5 OR MORE (EACH SIDE)   REST: 0 SEC.

Get into pushup position resting your left hand on the medicine ball and right hand on the floor. Lower your body until your chest is just above the floor and then push back up. At the top, reach up with your opposite hand and slap your chest.

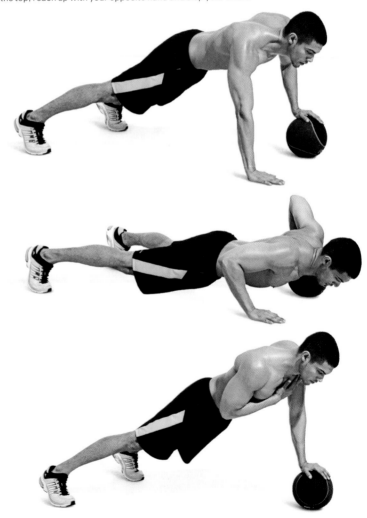

2 DROP N' POP

SETS: 1-3   REPS: 5 OR MORE   REST: 0 SEC.

Place both hands on the ball and get into pushup position. Quickly let go of the ball and spread your hands out to shoulder width on the floor. When you feel your chest touch the ball, push yourself up fast so your hands come off the floor and land on the ball again.

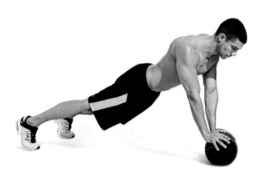

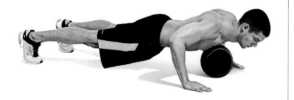

3 CLOSE-GRIP PUSHUP

SETS: 1-3   REPS: 5 OR MORE   REST: 0 SEC.

With both hands on the ball, perform pushups. Squeeze the ball hard throughout the set and keep your abs braced.

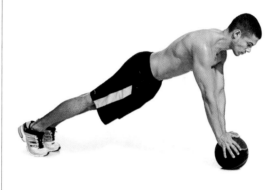

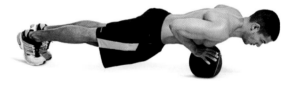

4 CROSSOVER PUSHUP

SETS: 1-3   REPS: 5 OR MORE   REST: 3-5 MINUTES

Perform a pushup with one hand on the ball, then quickly switch hands and do another rep.

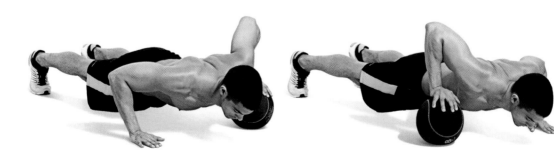

THE BEST BAND-ONLY CHEST WORKOUT

WORKOUT #45   BY JIM SMITH, C.S.C.S.

One of the best ways to make a muscle grow is to make it stretch at the bottom of a rep. This helps recruit muscle fibers and signals the nervous system that it needs to contract hard to prevent any further stretching, which could cause injury. Bands are great for feeling a stretch on chest exercises and, combined with pushups, can pump your pecs up fast.

HOW IT WORKS The chest can get worked in every way, even when heavy weights aren't available. The plyo pushup recruits some of the strongest pec fibers, and band flyes and pushups stretch and exhaust them from a variety of angles. Be prepared to walk out of the gym so pumped that your chest passes through the doorway long before your chin does.

DIRECTIONS Perform the paired exercises (marked "A" and "B") as supersets. So you'll do one set of A and then B before resting. Complete all the prescribed sets for the pair before moving on. The last exercise is done with conventional straight sets.

1A PLYO PUSHUP

SETS: 4   REPS: 6-8   REST: 0 SEC.

Perform pushups, but explode upward on each rep so that your hands leave the floor and you can clap before landing. When you land, go immediately into the next rep. Stop the set as soon as your movement slows down, even if it's before six reps are completed.

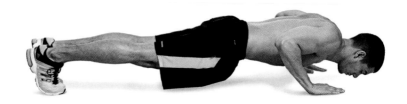
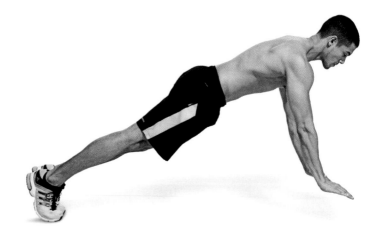

1B WIDE-GRIP PUSHUP

SETS: 4   REPS: 20   REST: 90-120 SEC.

Place your hands wider than shoulder width and perform pushups.

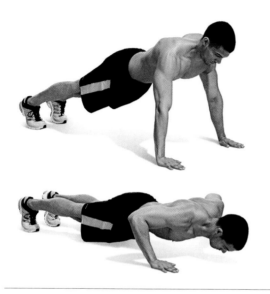

2A BAND-RESISTED PUSHUP W/ FEET ELEVATED

SETS: 4   REPS: 8-10   REST: 0 SEC.

Grasp an end of the band in one hand and wrap it around your back. Pin both hands to the floor with the ends of the band in your palms. Rest your feet on a box, bench, or mats so that your body forms a straight line parallel to the floor. Perform pushups.

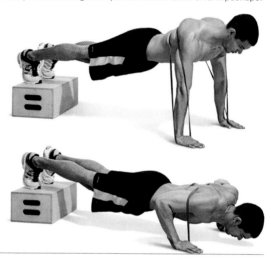

2B BAND-RESISTED FLYE

SETS: 4   REPS: AS MANY AS POSSIBLE   REST: 90 SEC.

Attach a band to a sturdy object at shoulder height and repeat with another adjacent to it. Or wrap a band around the object and hold an end in each hand. Step forward so that your arms are drawn back 90 degrees to your sides and you feel a stretch in your pecs. Keeping your elbows slightly bent, bring your hands together in front of your chest as if you were giving someone a bear hug.

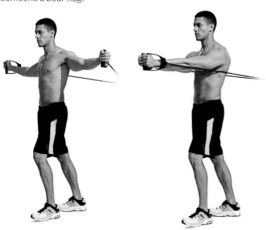

3 PUSHUP

SETS: AS MANY AS NEEDED   REPS: 150 TOTAL

Perform 150 total reps, taking as many sets as you need and resting as little as possible between them. If pushups are easy for you, begin using the band for resistance and then get rid of it as fatigue sets in and finish your reps with body weight alone.

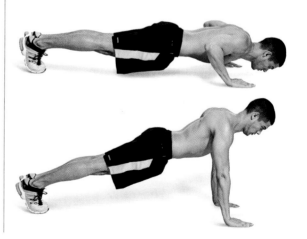

THE BEST BODY-WEIGHT CHEST WORKOUT

WORKOUT #46   BY BEN BRUNO

The chest is probably the easiest muscle group to build up when you have no equipment. All you really need is the trusty pushup to do it. Too many guys get bored of pushups and think they can graduate to the bench press, but if you can't do 100 reps in a handful of sets, your pecs aren't as strong as they could be and you're missing out on gains that are easily gotten through body-weight training alone.

HOW IT WORKS This workout is all about the pushup—doing it and helping you do it better in future training sessions. You'll work to get 100 total reps in as few sets as possible, and then strengthen your triceps and core directly. These muscles support your ability to do pushups, so the stronger they are, the more pushups you can crank out and the bigger your chest will get.

Simple enough.

DIRECTIONS Perform the pushups as conventional straight sets. Perform the exercise pairs (marked "A" and "B") as alternating sets. So you'll do a set of A, rest, then a set of B, rest again, and continue for all the prescribed sets.

1 PUSHUP

SETS: AS MANY AS NEEDED   REPS: 100 TOTAL   REST: AS NEEDED

Perform pushups, but go one rep shy of failure on each set and try to complete 100 reps in as few sets as possible. When you can do it in fewer than five sets, increase the number to 120 total reps.

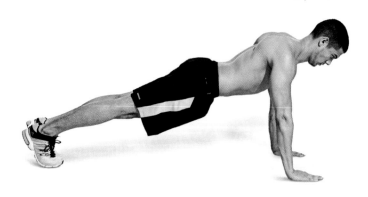

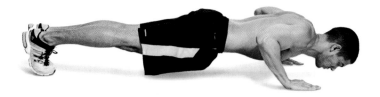

2A TRICEPS EXTENSION

SETS: 3   REPS: 12   REST: 90 SEC.

Start in pushup position and then rest your forearms on the floor with palms down. Keeping your core tight and your body in a straight line, extend your elbows so your arms are straight.

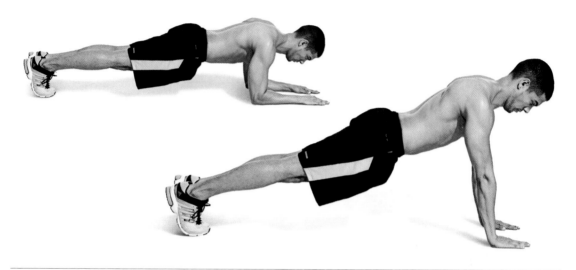

2B PLANK

SETS: 3   REPS: HOLD FOR 60 SEC.   REST: 60 SEC.

Get into pushup position and bend your elbows to lower your forearms to the floor. Hold the position with abs braced.

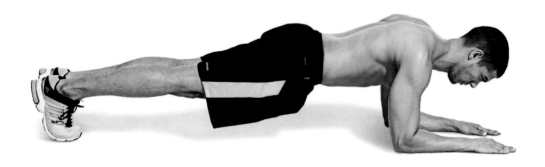

17 **SHOULDERS**

The shoulder joints are especially mobile and, as a result, are prime candidates for injury, especially if you bench heavy. Our shoulder workouts take into account weaknesses and imbalances you're probably already suffering (whether you know it or not) to prevent you from hurting something that might take months to fix. If your shoulders already bother you, you'll find that some of our exercises allow you to keep building them up without aggravating any injury, and may even correct the problem along the way.

THE BEST
FULL-GYM SHOULDER WORKOUT

WORKOUT #47   BY LEE BOYCE, C.P.T.

With access to all that a gym has to offer, you can work your shoulders from a variety of angles and, while you're at it, rep schemes. Lower reps (six and under) with heavy weights result in the best strength gains. Medium reps (8-12) with moderate loads exhaust the muscles, sparking gains in sheer size. High reps (15 or more) train endurance, but in so doing hit a different set of muscle fibers that aren't tapped by the other rep ranges. The shoulder routine here takes advantage of all three ranges to leave no stone unturned in your journey for bigger delts.

HOW IT WORKS The exercises are organized into trisets—three moves done back to back. The first lift in each triset is done heavy, the second is medium, and the third is light but for high reps. Combine the variety of the exercises, the rep ranges, and the fast pace and there's little more you can do to shock your delts into new growth.

DIRECTIONS Perform the first triset (marked as "A," "B," and "C") in sequence without rest in between. Afterward, rest two to three minutes, and repeat for four total trisets. Then go on to the second triset and complete it in the same fashion.

1A OVERHEAD PRESS

SETS: 4 REPS: 6 REST: 0 SEC.

Set the bar up in a squat rack or cage, and grasp it just outside shoulder width. Take the bar off the rack and hold it at shoulder level with your forearms perpendicular to the floor. Squeeze the bar and brace your abs. Press the bar overhead, pushing your head forward and shrugging your traps as the bar passes your face.

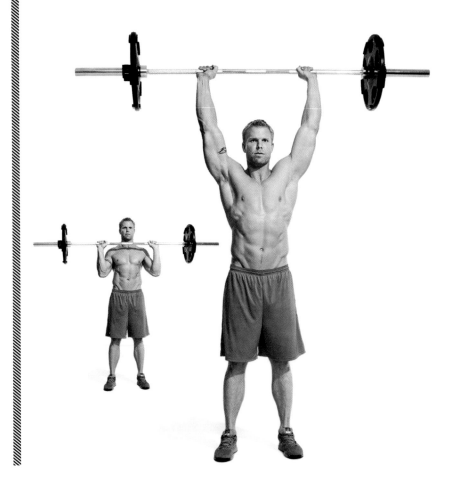

1B STANDING DUMBBELL FLYE

SETS: 4   REPS: 12   REST: 0 SEC.

Hold a dumbbell in each hand by your sides. Without shrugging, use your upper body to swing the weights up a few inches. Your arms and torso will form an upside down V shape. Think of it as a lateral raise with momentum but without full range of motion.

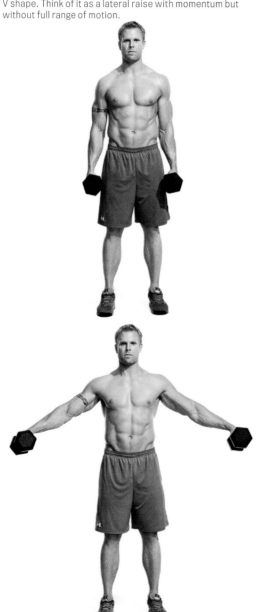

1C FACE PULL

SETS: 4   REPS: 25   REST: 120-180 SEC.

Attach a rope handle to the top pulley of a cable station. Grasp an end in each hand with palms facing each other. Step back to place tension on the cable. Pull the handles to your forehead so your palms face your ears and your upper back is fully contracted.

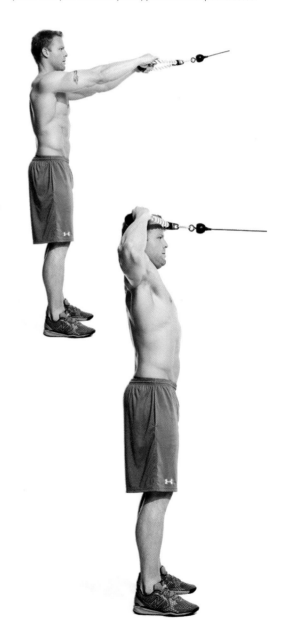

2A HIGH PULL

SETS: 4   REPS: 6   REST: 0 SEC.

Grasp the bar with hands about double shoulder width and hold it in front of your thighs. Bend your knees and hips so the bar hangs just above your knees. Explosively extend your hips as if jumping and pull the bar up to shoulder level with elbows wide apart, as in an upright row.

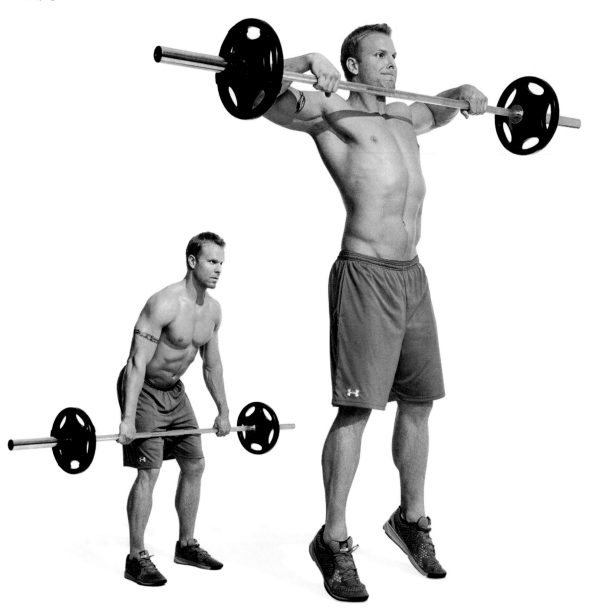

2B SEATED DUMBBELL CLEAN

SETS: 4   REPS: 12   REST: 0 SEC.

Hold a dumbbell in each hand and sit on the edge of a bench. Keeping your lower back flat, lean forward. Explosively straighten your body and shrug the weights so your arms rise. Allow the momentum to flip your wrists so you catch the weights at shoulder level.

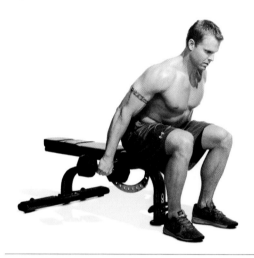
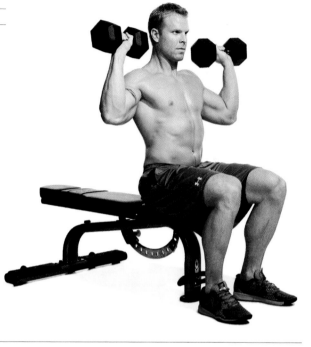

2C TRAP RAISE

SETS: 4   REPS: 25   REST: 120-180 SEC.

Set a bench to a low incline and lie chest-down with a dumbbell in each hand and your palms facing. Retract your shoulder blades, then raise the weights straight out so your arms are parallel to the floor.

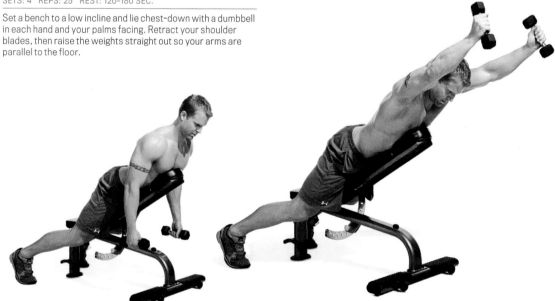

THE BEST BARBELL-ONLY SHOULDER WORKOUT

WORKOUT #48   BY JASON FERRUGGIA

Olympic weightlifters typically have big, broad shoulders, and they use barbells almost exclusively in their training. The deltoid muscles simply don't need a lot of training variety if you're regularly exploding big weights off the ground and overhead. This workout incorporates weightlifting movements to build your delts, but don't be disappointed if other muscles happen to get bigger and stronger, too.

HOW IT WORKS The clean and press is frequently called the most functional exercise of all, because it works every last muscle in your body to perform a basic movement pattern—picking something up and raising it overhead. The high pull isn't done with heavy weights, but the speed you perform it at recruits all the biggest and strongest muscle fibers. Note that we're also having you perform it with an extra-wide snatch grip. This makes the move easier on your shoulder joints, so you don't inadvertently break them while you're trying to build the muscle that surrounds them.

DIRECTIONS Complete all sets for the clean and press and then move on to the snatch-grip high pull.

1 CLEAN AND PRESS

SETS: 4   REPS: 6–8   REST: 90 SEC.

Stand with feet shoulder width. Keeping your lower back arched, bend your hips back to lower your torso and grasp the bar with hands shoulder width. Extend your hips to lift the bar off the floor. When it gets past your knees, jump and shrug the bar so that momentum raises it and you catch it at shoulder level. Brace your abs and stand tall. Press the bar straight overhead.

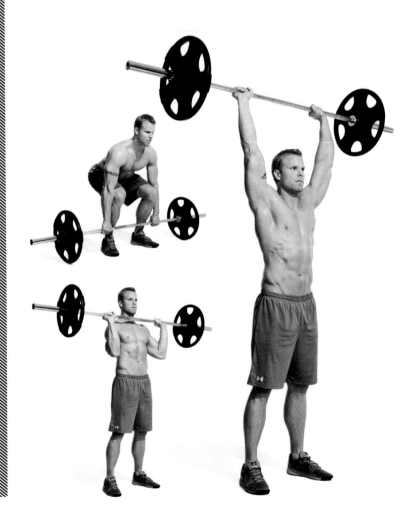

2 SNATCH-GRIP HIGH PULL

SETS: 4   REPS: 6   REST: 90 SEC.

Set up as you did for the clean and press, but grasp the bar with hands double shoulder width. Explode the bar upward until it's at chest level and your upper arms are parallel to the floor. Try to push your chest out as you lift the bar and contract your upper back completely.

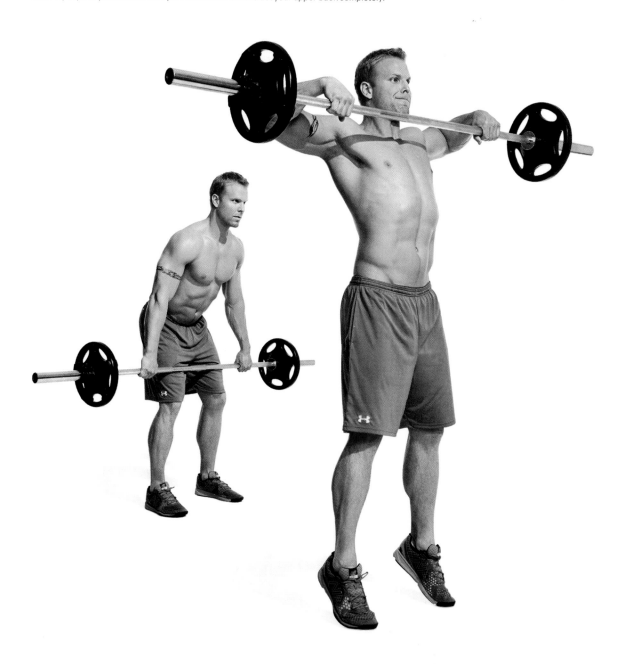

THE BEST BAND-ONLY SHOULDER WORKOUT

WORKOUT #49   BY JIM SMITH, C.S.C.S.

The knock on lateral raises done with free weights is that the first half of the movement is easy. Your shoulders only start to really kick in toward the top, when your arms are extended out from your sides. Bands, however, put tension on your muscles throughout the whole movement and make it harder at the end range of motion. If you thought bands were just making the best of a bad situation (no free weights), this workout will change your mind—and fry your shoulders.

HOW IT WORKS We've taken conventional free-weight shoulder exercises like the overhead press, lateral raise, and shrug and applied bands to them. You'll have to fight the resistance on each movement as it increases, which heightens the demand on your muscles and also teaches you to lift fast. If you can't explode your reps, you won't be able to lock them out, so you have to do your sets deliberately and with power; and power training recruits the biggest muscle fibers.

DIRECTIONS Perform the exercises marked with letters in sequence. For instance, for pairs of "A" and "B" exercises, you'll do a set of A and then B before resting. Repeat until all sets are completed. For exercises 2A, 2B, and 2C, perform all three in order before resting and then repeat. The first exercise (overhead press) is done as straight sets.

1 OVERHEAD PRESS

SETS: 4   REPS: 6-8   REST: 60 SEC.

Stand on the middle of a band (or use two, depending on the length) and hold an end in each hand at shoulder level. Stand tall with glutes and abs braced, and press overhead.

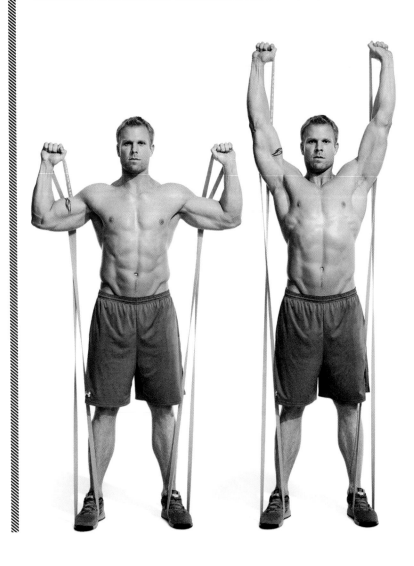

2A LATERAL RAISE

SETS: 3 REPS: 12-15 REST: 0 SEC.

Step on the free end of each band with the opposite foot so the bands form an X in front of your body. Raise your arms 90 degrees out to the sides until your upper arms are parallel to the floor.

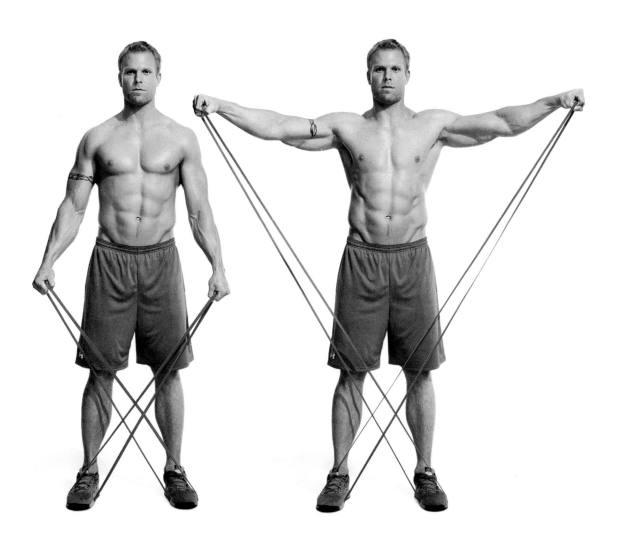

2B FRONT RAISE

SETS: 3   REPS: 12–15   REST: 0 SEC.

Stand on bands and hold the opposite ends. Raise your arms in front of your body to shoulder height.

2C BENTOVER LATERAL RAISE

SETS: 3   REPS: 12–15   REST: 90 SEC.

Stand on the end of one band with your right foot and hold it with your left hand. Do the opposite with another band so that the bands cross each other. Bend your hips back until your torso is almost parallel to the floor. The bands should be taut in this starting position. Squeeze your shoulder blades together and raise your arms out to your sides.

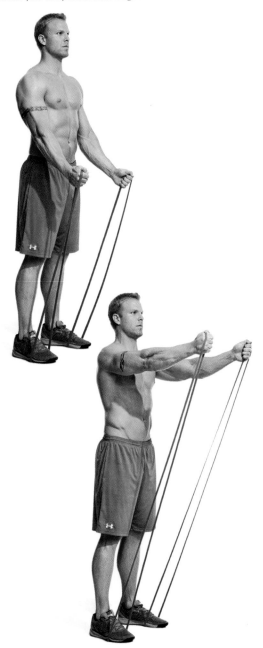

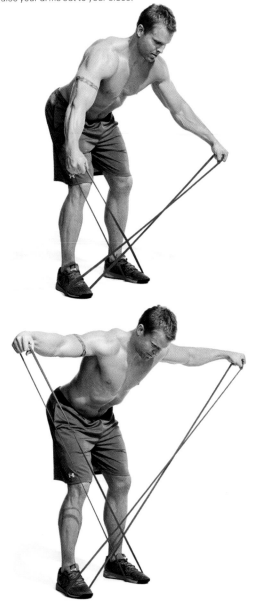

3A SHRUG

SETS: 3   REPS: 20   REST: 0 SEC.

Stand on the middle of a band and grasp an end with arms by your sides. Standing tall, shrug your shoulders to your ears.

3B W RAISE

SETS: 3   REPS: 20   REST: 60 SEC.

Attach bands to a sturdy object at shoulder level and hold the opposite ends in each hand. Stand back to put tension on the bands. Squeeze your shoulder blades together and row the bands to your shoulders with elbows flared out so your upper arms make a W shape. Hold for two seconds.

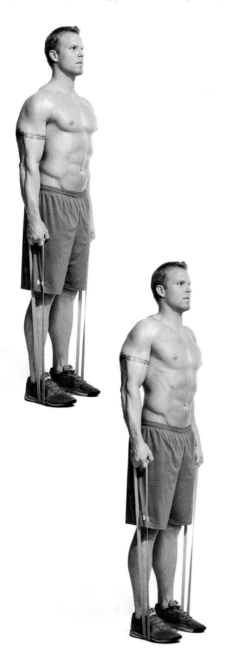

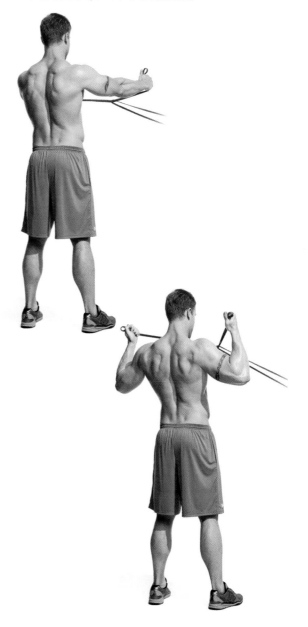

THE BEST SUSPENSION-TRAINER SHOULDER WORKOUT

WORKOUT #50   BY JASON FERRUGGIA

The following suspension trainer workout helps target the rear delts, a muscle group that is generally underutilized and, as a consequence, underdeveloped. The imbalance results from sitting at desks with poor posture for hours on end and is compounded by most gymgoers' preference for bench presses over rear-delt exercises.

This workout forces your rear delts to work harder than they ever have, and you'll need only your body weight to do it.

HOW IT WORKS The Y raise and rear-delt flye may be familiar to you, as they're often performed with dumbbells. But a suspension trainer makes them more effective because you're lifting your body weight as opposed to tiny (and possibly pink) hand weights. Obviously, this activates more muscle, and makes you look more like a gymnast than an old lady in her first personal training session.

DIRECTIONS Complete all the sets for one move before going on to the next.

1 PIKE PUSHUP

SETS: 4   REPS: 8-12   REST: 90 SEC.

Attach the suspension trainer to a sturdy object overhead, and lower the foot cradles to about knee height (you want your body to be in a straight line when you rest your feet in them). Get into pushup position with your feet in the cradles and hands placed shoulder width on the floor. Keeping your abs braced, lower your body until your chest is just above the floor and then push back up. Now bend your hips and raise them into the air until your torso is vertical. Straighten your body again. That's one rep.

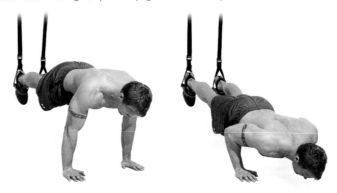

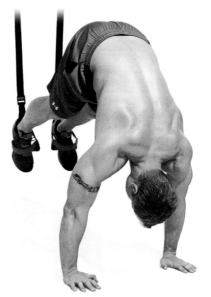

2 Y RAISE

SETS: 2   REPS: 12-15   REST: 60 SEC.

Grasp the handles and stand with feet about shoulder width. Lean back 45–60 degrees, so your body is supported by the trainer, and brace your abs. Raise your arms up and out into a Y shape with palms facing forward. Your body will become more vertical, but don't allow your shoulders to lose tension at the top of the movement. Your weight will shift from the back foot to the front foot.

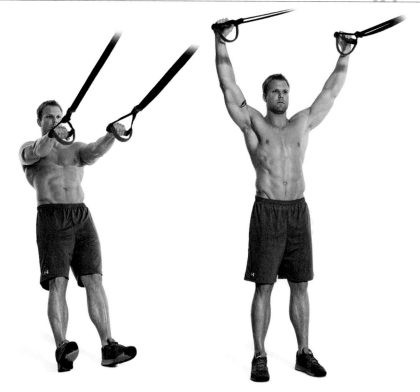

3 REAR-DELT FLYE

SETS: 4   REPS: 12-15   REST: 60 SEC.

Shorten the length of the handles, but stand as you did for the Y raise. Open your arms out to your sides with palms facing in until your shoulder blades are squeezed together. Allow a little bend in your elbows.

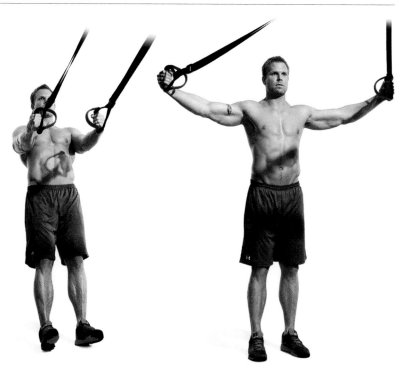

THE BEST BODY-WEIGHT SHOULDER WORKOUT

WORKOUT #51   BY JIM SMITH, C.S.C.S.

Muscles need tension to grow, and whether they get it from weights or your own body doesn't matter. When the tension is strong enough, and lasts long enough, your muscles will be forced to adapt by growing bigger and stronger. This workout uses trisets to supply the time and some brutally challenging body-weight movements to induce the tension.

HOW IT WORKS Trisets are tough. You do one exercise and then another and then another before you get to rest. This keeps your shoulders working a long time, and with these exercises, they're working to support your body in awkard positions where you're lifting large percentages of your own weight. You won't miss your dumbbells. At the end of each triset is a stretch, which encourages blood flow to the muscles, resulting in more nutrient delivery that helps them grow.

DIRECTIONS Perform exercises 1A, 1B, and 1C as a triset. So you'll complete one set of A, then B, and then C before resting. Repeat until all the prescribed sets are done, and then do exercises 2A, 2B, and 2C in the same fashion. Exercise 3 is performed with conventional straight sets.

1A HINDU PUSHUP

SETS: 4   REPS: 12-15   REST: 0 SEC.

Get into pushup position. Push your hands into the floor to drive your weight back so your hips rise into the air. Your back should be straight and your head behind your hands. Lower your body in an arcing motion so that your chest scoops downward and nearly scrapes the floor. Continue moving forward as you press your body up so your torso is vertical and your legs are straight and nearly on the floor. That's one rep.

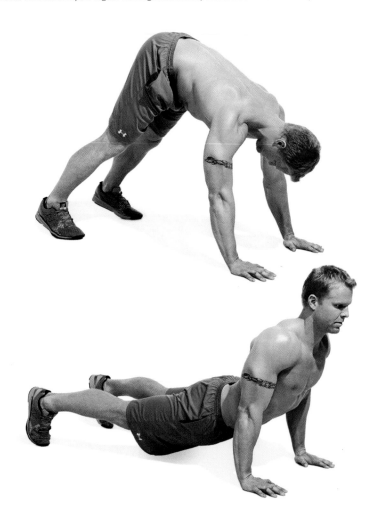

1B Y TO W RAISE

SETS: 4   REPS: 12-15   REST: 0 SEC.

Lie facedown on the floor and raise your arms overhead and out to your sides a bit with thumbs facing the ceiling. Your arms should form a Y shape with your body. Hold for a second. From there, bend your elbows and draw your arms back until your elbows are near your sides and your body now forms a W shape. Hold for a second. Think about doing a pullup—you're performing the same movement on the floor.

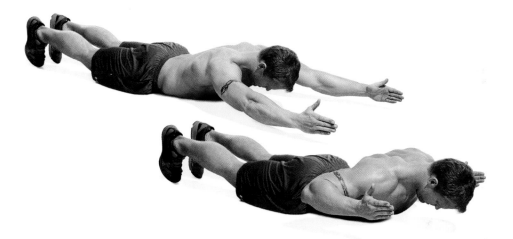

1C SHOULDER STRETCH

SETS: 4   REPS: HOLD FOR 30 SEC. (EACH SIDE)
REST: 30 SEC.

Place the inner side of your forearm against a doorframe with your elbow bent 90 degrees. Gently turn your torso away so you feel a stretch in your shoulder and pec muscles.

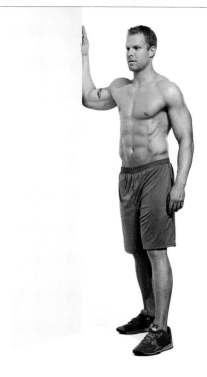

2A PIKE PRESS

SETS: 4   REPS: 8-10   REST: 0 SEC.

Get into pushup position and push your hips back so your torso is nearly vertical. Your hands, arms, and head should be in a straight line. Lower your body until your head nearly touches the floor between your hands and then press back up.

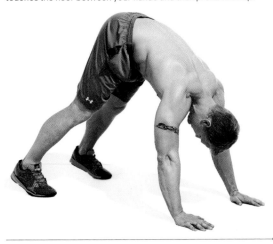 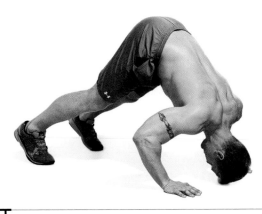

2B DIP

SETS: 4   REPS: 12-15   REST: 0 SEC.

Rest the palms of your hands on a bench or chair, and, if available, place your heels on another elevated object in front of you so your legs are suspended. Lower your body until your upper arms are parallel to the floor.

2C LAT STRETCH

SETS: 4   REPS/TIME: HOLD FOR 30 SEC. (EACH SIDE)   REST: 30 SEC.

Grasp a doorknob or other sturdy object at approximately the same level and bend your hips back, keeping your lower back flat, until your arm is in line with your torso. Rock your hips side to side so you feel a stretch in your lat muscle.

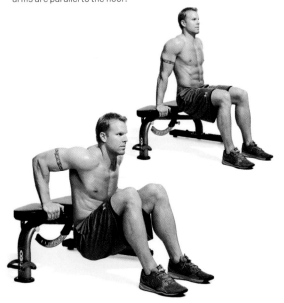 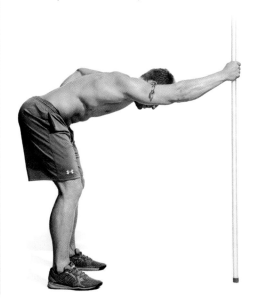

3 LATERAL PLANK WALK

SETS: 4 REPS: 10 SHUFFLES (EACH
WAY) REST: 60 SEC.

Get into pushup position and
simultaneously move your left hand
over your right while your right leg
steps out wide. Now bring the right
hand out and walk your left foot in
to a normal pushup footing. That's
one shuffle. Continue "walking"
for 10 shuffles and then walk in the
opposite direction to get back to
the starting position. Keep your
core braced and your hips level at
all times.

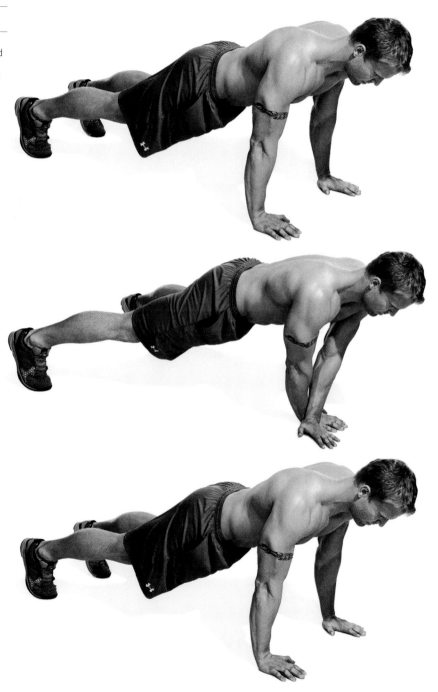

THE BEST DUMBBELL-ONLY SHOULDER WORKOUT

WORKOUT #52   BY C.J. MURPHY, M.F.S.

Your average trainer can think of only two ways to work your shoulders with dumbbells—presses and raises. We've got a third to add to the mix, and this three-pronged attack can build shoulders as round and dense as cannonballs.

HOW IT WORKS The first exercise, a neutral-grip over-head press, is the safest way to do any pressing movement. If you've backed off of shoulder work in the past because it hurt to execute, relief can be as simple as turning your palms to face each other. In this position, your upper-arm bones can glide through the shoulder joints without risk of impingement.

You'll follow this up with a variety of shoulder raises, ending with a crucifix hold, in which you keep your arms raised for time. This is an exercise popular among strongman competitors, whose shoulders are the size of pumpkins. Finally, the workout ends with seated dumbbell cleans. If you've ever done power cleans, you know what exploding a weight up from the floor to shoulder level can do for your shoulders, and this variation isolates them more. It's as simple to do as it sounds: heave the weights up. Brute force builds big shoulders.

DIRECTIONS Complete all sets for one exercise before moving on to the next.

1 NEUTRAL-GRIP OVERHEAD PRESS

SETS: 5   REPS: 8   REST: 60 SEC.

Hold a dumbbell in each hand at shoulder level with palms facing each other and elbows pointing forward. Brace your core and press the weights straight overhead. At the top, shrug your shoulders and hold for a second.

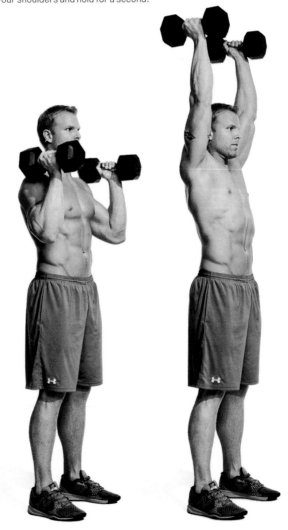

2 RAISE COMPLEX

SETS: 3   REPS: 12–15
REST: SEE BELOW

Hold dumbbells at your sides with palms facing you. Raise the weights up in front of you to shoulder level with thumbs pointing up. Complete 12–15 reps and then raise the weights out to your sides 90 degrees (bend your elbows a bit as you lift). Complete your reps and then switch to a lighter pair of dumbbells. Raise them out to your sides and up to ear level with straight arms and thumbs pointing up. Hold this position 30 seconds. Squeeze your glutes to help support you.

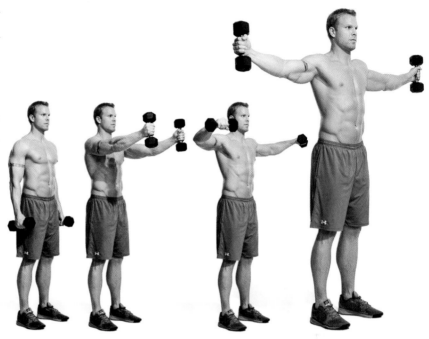

3 SEATED DUMBBELL CLEAN

SETS: 3   REPS: 12–15   REST: 60 SEC.

Hold a dumbbell in each hand and sit on the edge of a bench. Keeping your lower back flat, lean forward. Explosively straighten your body and shrug the weights so your arms rise. Allow the momentum to flip your wrists so you catch the weights at shoulder level.

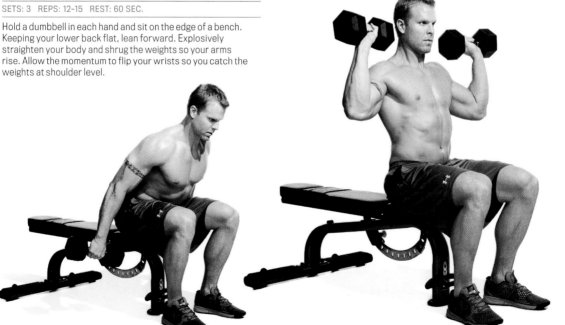

18

BACK

Getting your mind into back training isn't as easy as it is with the chest and arms. Because you can't see your back, it is tougher to visualize how it is working, and so you must learn to focus on the feeling of your muscles contracting with each rep. Finding the right training implements for your needs can help with this. If dumbbells don't work for you, bands might, because their accommodating resistance makes reps feel different than with free weights. It's possible that simple pullups do the trick, because you're able to imagine your hands as hooks designed to allow your lats to move your body up and down. Whatever may work best for you, we've got it covered here, so you can build your back with the same intensity you do your arms.

THE BEST
FULL-GYM BACK WORKOUT

WORKOUT #53   BY JIM SMITH, C.S.C.S.

Deadlifts are one of our favorite exercises at *Men's Fitness*. They raise testosterone, jack up your metabolism, and add slabs of muscle all over your body–and to your back in particular. Deadlifts are the centerpiece of this routine, and just when they've worn you out, the work really begins.

HOW IT WORKS The deadlift is a strenuous exercise and usually requires plenty of rest between sets. No such luck here. You'll keep your rest periods short and squeak out as many reps as you can to exhaust your back completely. Then you'll go on to chinups– the ultimate lat builder–lying lateral raises, rows, and back extensions. To tell you the truth, the deadlift alone will leave your back sore the next morning. The rest of the exercises just keep it that way longer.

DIRECTIONS Perform the paired exercises (marked "A" and "B") as supersets. So you'll do one set of A and then B before resting. Complete all the prescribed sets for the pair before moving on. The first exercise is done as conventional straight sets.

1 DEADLIFT

SETS: 4 REPS: 5, AS MANY AS POSSIBLE REST: 15 SEC.

Stand with feet hip width and bend your hips back to grasp the bar just outside your knees. Keeping your back flat, extend your hips to stand up, pulling the bar up along your legs to lockout. Perform three warmup sets of five reps using 20%, 40%, and 60% of your deadlift max, respectively. (If you don't know how much you can lift for one rep on the deadlift, estimate it conservatively.) Rest 90 seconds between these warmups. When you're done, perform one set with 70-75% of your max for five reps and then rest 15 seconds. Perform three more sets of as many reps as possible, resting 15 seconds between sets. You may get only one or two reps on these last three sets, and that's OK. End a set if you suspect your form might be compromised.

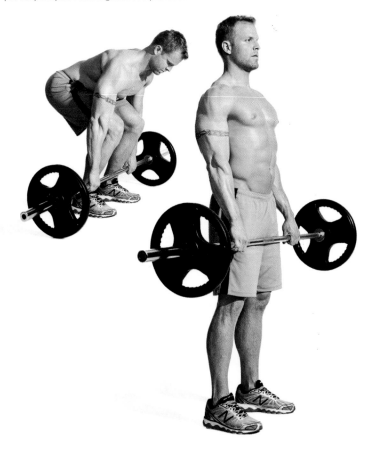

2A CHINUP

SETS: 4 REPS: 6-8 REST: 0 SEC.

Hang from a chinup bar with hands shoulder width. Pull yourself up until your chin is over the bar.

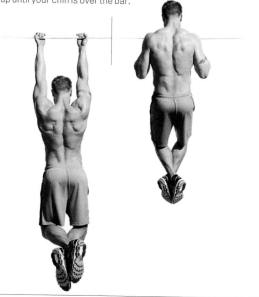

2B LYING LATERAL RAISE

SETS: 4 REPS: 20 REST: 60-90 SEC.

Set an adjustable bench to a 30-degree incline and lie on it chest-down with a dumbbell in each hand. Squeeze your shoulder blades together and raise your arms out 90 degrees to your sides so your palms face down in the top position.

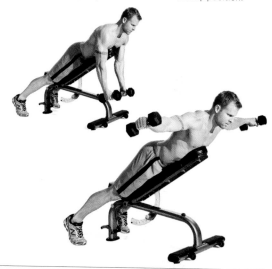

3A SEATED CABLE ROW

SETS: 3 REPS: 10-12 REST: 0 SEC.

Attach a straight or lat-pulldown bar to the pulley of a seated row station. Sit on the bench (or floor) with your feet against the foot plate and knees slightly bent. Keeping your lower back flat, bend forward at the hips to grasp the bar and row it to your sternum, squeezing your shoulder blades together in the end position. Extend your arms and feel the stretch in your back before beginning the next rep.

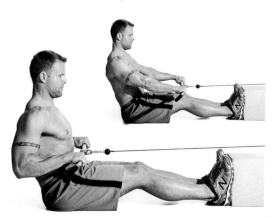

3B BACK EXTENSION

SETS: 3 REPS: 10-12 REST: 60 SEC.

Lock your legs into a back extension bench and allow your torso to bend forward so that your hips are bent almost 90 degrees. Extend your hips so that your body forms a straight line.

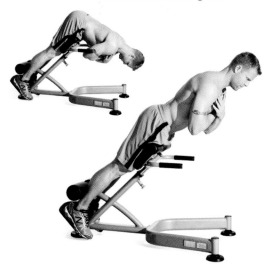

THE BEST BARBELL-ONLY BACK WORKOUT

WORKOUT #54   BY JASON FERRUGGIA

People who train mainly with barbells never seem to lack back development. Regardless of what exercises you do to target other muscles–Olympic lifts, squats, or deadlifts–just holding and stabilizing the bar places a demand on everything from the traps down to the spinal erectors. This barebones routine will thicken you front to back and widen you side to side.

HOW IT WORKS You'll begin with the hang clean, an Olympic weightlifting exercise that works everything but requires the traps to help heave weights from the knees to the shoulders. Then you can target the lats with rows from various angles. If overemphasizing chest work has left your front and back out of balance, you couldn't ask for a better tool than the trusty barbell to set things right.

DIRECTIONS Complete all sets for one exercise before going on to the next.

1 HANG CLEAN

SETS: 3   REPS: 6   REST: 90 SEC.

Hold the bar at shoulder width in front of your thighs and bend your hips and knees so that the bar lowers to just above your knees. Now explosively extend your hips as if jumping while at the same time shrugging your shoulders and pulling the bar straight up in front of your torso. As the bar reaches chest level, bend your elbows and flip your wrists to catch the bar at shoulder level, palms face the ceiling. Bend your hips and knees as you catch the bar to absorb the impact.

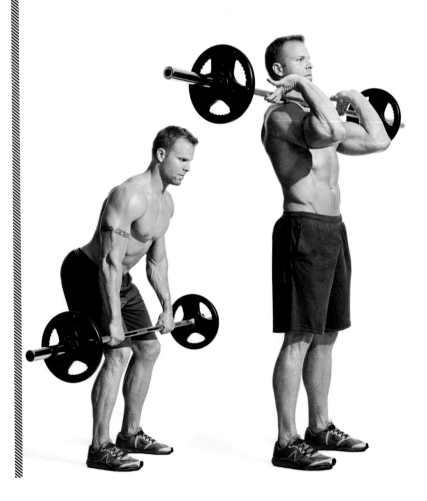

2 LANDMINE ONE-ARM ROW

SETS: 3   REPS: 12, 10, 8 (EACH SIDE)   REST: 90 SEC.

Wedge the end of the bar into a corner (you may have to wrap it in a towel to protect the walls). Face away from the corner and hold the barbell behind the sleeve (where you load the weights) with your right hand. Stagger your legs so that your left leg is forward and, keeping your lower back flat, bend at the hips until your torso is about parallel to the floor. Draw your shoulder blade back and row the bar to your ribs.

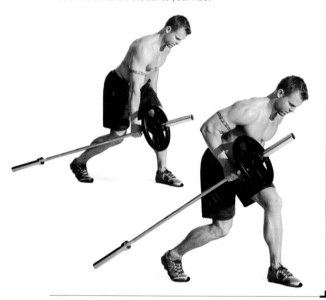

3 YATES ROW

SETS: 2   REPS: 10-12   REST: 90 SEC.

Hold the bar with an underhand grip at shoulder width. Keeping your lower back in its natural arch, bend your hips back and lower your torso to about 60 degrees. Row the weight to your belly button using a slight cheat (use momentum to begin each rep), but don't let your lower back round. If you have wrist straps, you may use them to help your grip.

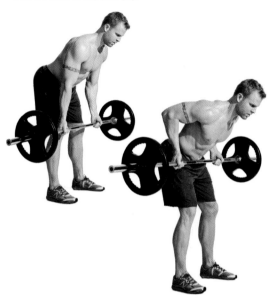

4 BENTOVER ROW TO NECK

SETS: 2   REPS: 12-15   REST: 60 SEC.

Set up as you did for the Yates row, but grasp the bar overhand and bend forward more until your torso is parallel to the floor. Squeeze your shoulder blades together and row the weight to your neck. Note that you'll have to use light weights.

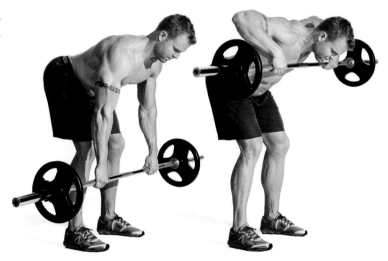

THE BEST DUMBBELL-ONLY BACK WORKOUT

WORKOUT #55   BY MICHAEL SCHLETTER, C.P.T.

The lower back takes a beating in most strength exercises. If you're the type who likes to squat, deadlift, and overhead press a lot, you know how sore that area can get even when you feel your other muscles are doing all the work. In this routine, we train it both directly and indirectly to fortify it for all future workouts, while training your lats hard at the same time.

HOW IT WORKS You'll spend most of the workout staring at the floor. That's because you'll be bent over holding the arch in your lower back while giving your main attention to your lats and rear delts. This will teach these muscles to act synergistically and keep your spine protected for future heavy rows, deadlifts, and so on. The stronger your lower back, the more weight you can handle on most other exercises (not just for back), and greater loads mean bigger muscles.

DIRECTIONS Perform the paired exercises (marked "A" and "B") as supersets. So you'll do one set of A and then B before resting. Complete all the prescribed sets for the pair before moving on. The last exercise is done as conventional straight sets.

1A ONE-ARM NEUTRAL-GRIP ROW

SETS: 5 REPS: 5-8 (EACH SIDE) REST: SEE BELOW

Hold a dumbbell in one hand and, keeping your lower back in its natural arch, bend your hips back until your torso is parallel to the floor and your arm is hanging down with your thumb pointing forward. Draw your shoulder blade back and row the weight to your side. After you complete your set on both sides, start a timer for three minutes, and go on to 1B.

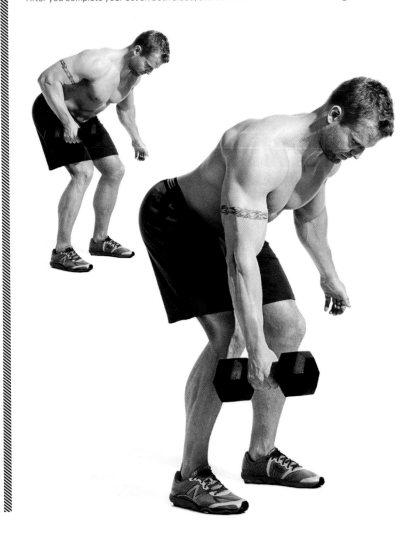

1B BENTOVER REVERSE FLYE

SETS: 5 REPS: 10-12 REST: 3 MIN.

Set up as you did for the neutral-grip row but with lighter dumbbells. Raise your arms out to your sides 90 degrees, squeezing your shoulder blades together at the top for a second. Complete your set and then rest until the end of three minutes, when your timer goes off.

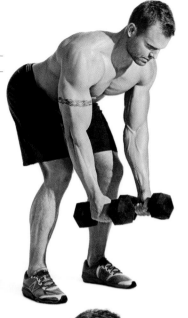

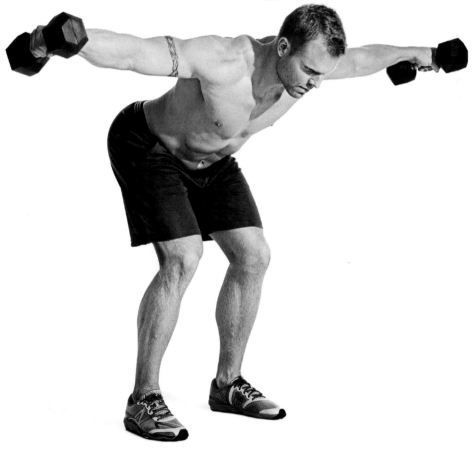

2A ONE-ARM UNDERHAND ROW

SETS: 3 REPS: 8-12 (EACH SIDE) REST: 0 SEC.

From the same bentover starting position, turn your palm to face in front of you and row the weight to your side.

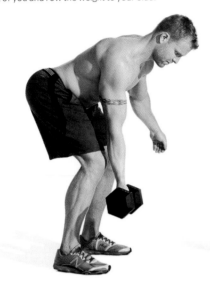
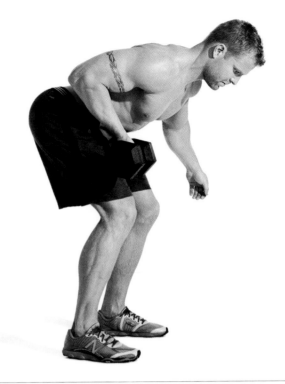

2B PRONE BACK EXTENSION

SETS: 3 REPS: 12-15 REST: 120 SEC.

Lie facedown on the floor with arms extended by your sides. Raise your torso off the floor as high as you can and hold at the top for a second.

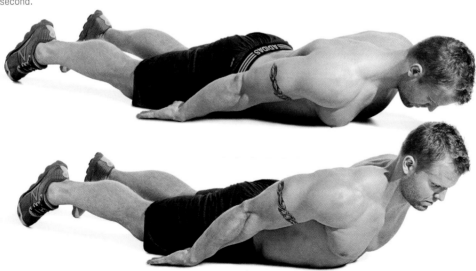

3A AQUAMAN

SETS: 4 REPS: AS MANY AS POSSIBLE (EACH SIDE) REST: 0 SEC.

Set up as you did for the back extension and then raise your left arm and right leg off the floor. Hold at the top for a second with both limbs straight and then lower back down.

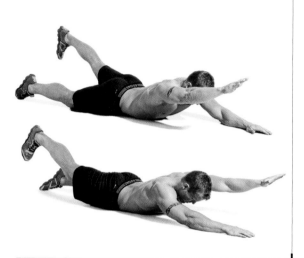

3B BENTOVER ROW

SETS: 4 REPS: 8-12 REST: 120 SEC.

Perform as you did the neutral-grip row, but use two dumbbells and turn your palms to face your thighs.

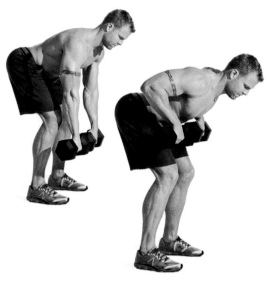

4 SUPERMAN

SETS: 2 REPS: HOLD FOR 20 SEC. REST: 60 SEC.

Perform as you did the back extension, but raise your hands and legs off the floor (and hold them straight) so that only your hips remain in contact with it.

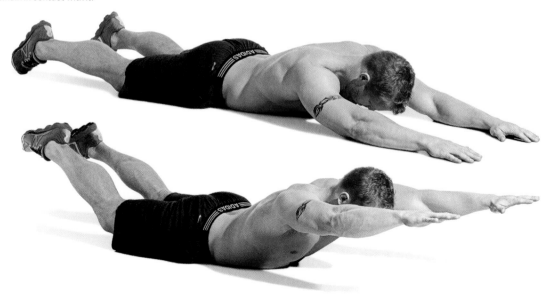

THE BEST SUSPENSION-TRAINER BACK WORKOUT

WORKOUT #56   BY BEN BRUNO

You know the expression that a chain is only as strong as its weakest link. Well, your muscles work like a chain, too. The smaller ones are weaker than the big ones and, thus, are more likely to "break," limiting the force the prime movers can produce and reducing the effectiveness of an exercise and your workout. If your back has stopped growing, it's time to start looking at the chain of muscles behind it, link by link.

HOW IT WORKS On any back exercise, the biceps and the rear head of the deltoid can't help but get involved. After all, they're pulling muscles too. But because they're smaller and weaker than your lats, they tend to hold back the weight you can use or the reps you can perform on exercises like rows and pullups. The routine at right incorporates shoulder and arm work, strengthening these areas so that they don't give out before your back does.

DIRECTIONS Perform the first two exercises as conventional straight sets. Perform the exercise pairs (marked "A" and "B") as alternating sets. So you'll do a set of A, rest, then a set of B, rest again, and continue for all the prescribed sets.

1 FLY-AWAY CHINUP

SETS: 3 REPS: 5 REST: 90 SEC.

Attach the suspension trainer to a sturdy object overhead and set the handles less than shoulder-width apart and high enough so that when you hang from them your feet will be off the floor. Grasp the handles with palms facing you and hang. Now pull yourself up until your chin is over your hands.

Begin to lower yourself, moving your elbows away from your body and rotating your palms to face forward. Do it slowly (it should take three to five seconds to come back down). That's one rep.

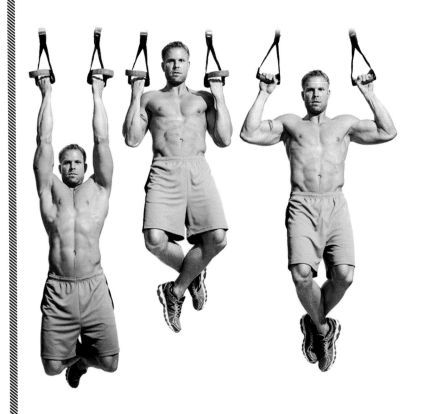

2 INVERTED ROW

SETS: SEE BELOW REPS: 75 TOTAL
REST: AS NEEDED

Lengthen the straps and hold the handles. Lean back with arms extended so that your body is supported by the trainer and only your feet are on the floor. Brace your core and hold your body in a straight line. (The lower you set the handles, the harder the exercise; you can elevate your feet on something to make it even harder.) With palms facing your feet, row your body up. Perform 75 total reps, resting as needed. Go one rep shy of failure each set.

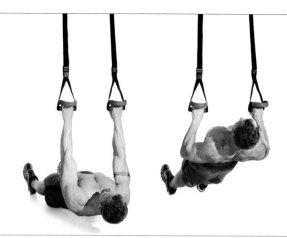

3A 3-WAY SHOULDER FINISHER

SETS: 3 REPS: 5 REST: 90 SEC.

Grasp the handles and lean back away from the trainer's attachment point so that your weight is on your heels and your body is about 45 degrees to the floor. Allow your arms to extend in front of you. Squeeze your shoulder blades together and draw your arms back until they're 90 degrees out to your sides. (Keep a slight bend in your elbows.) That's one rep of the reverse flye. Perform five reps.

Now, from the start position of the reverse flye, draw your upper arms back with your elbows bent 90 degrees and knuckles facing the ceiling. Your upper body should make a W shape. That's one rep of the external rotation. Perform five reps.

Return to the starting position with arms extended and pull your hands to your forehead, twisting your palms to face in front of you as you pull. That's one face pull. Perform five reps. All of the above equals one set.

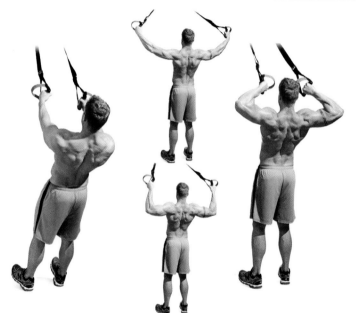

3B BICEPS CURL

SETS: 3 REPS: 10 REST: 90 SEC.

Face the trainer's attachment point and grasp the handles with palms facing up. Lean back with your abs braced, body straight, and arms extended in front of you. Curl your body up to the handles.

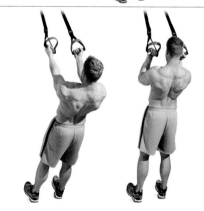

THE BEST BODY-WEIGHT BACK WORKOUT

WORKOUT #57   BY HARRY CLAY

Dropsets are when you take a set to failure and then immediately "drop" to a lighter weight and continue doing reps. Used sparingly, they're a smart way to increase intensity and extend a set past the point where you'd normally be spent. Most often, dropsets are done with dumbbells or machines, but your own body weight can be used for them too.

HOW IT WORKS The dropsets we're using work according to mechanical advantage. When your arms are spread wide apart, you don't have much leverage to pull yourself up, so wide-grip pullups are among the toughest of all pullup variations. The workout begins with those. When you've hit failure, it then goes to conventional chinups, which are easier.

When you can't do another chinup, you'll bring your hands even closer together, giving you the best mechanical advantage possible, and again rep out to failure. The trick is to keep the circuit going, switching to exercises that are just easy enough to let you continue doing reps. Unlike with weights, dropsets based on mechanical advantage allow you to keep the same load—your body—which ensures your lats get the greatest possible stimulus.

DIRECTIONS Perform the exercises as a circuit, completing one set of each in sequence without rest. Afterward, rest two minutes and then repeat the circuit once more.

1 WIDE-GRIP PULLUP

SETS: 2 REPS: AS MANY AS POSSIBLE REST: 0 SEC.

Grasp a pullup bar overhand and well outside shoulder width. Hang from the bar and then pull yourself up until your chin is over it. Complete your reps and then come down off the bar for a moment.

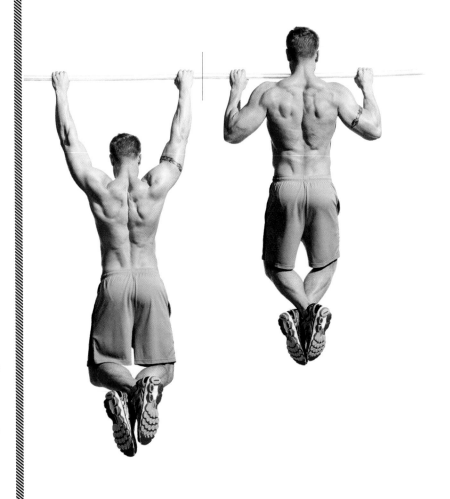

2 CHINUP

SETS: 2 REPS: AS MANY AS POSSIBLE REST: 0 SEC.

Grasp the bar with hands shoulder width and turn your palms to face you. Pull yourself up until your chin is over the bar. Complete your reps and then come down off the bar.

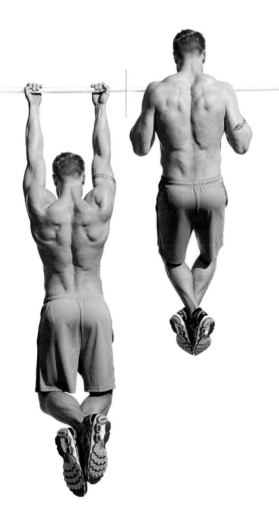

3 CLOSE-GRIP CHINUP

SETS: 2 REPS: AS MANY AS POSSIBLE REST: 120 SEC.

Grasp the bar with hands only six inches apart and palms facing you. Pull yourself up.

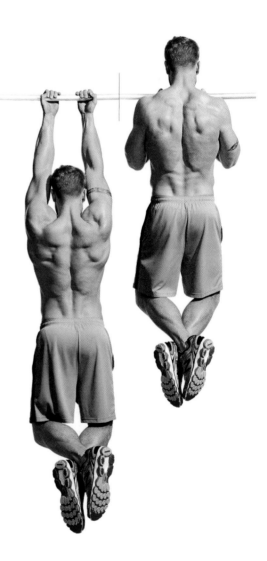

19

LEGS

You can't *not* train legs. Not only does it make you a wuss, but it holds back your gains in every other department. Because they're enormous muscles, working the legs causes greater release of natural anabolic hormones than any other body part. This contributes to the growth of all your muscles over time. And if you're interested in playing sports, running, and preventing a hip fracture when you're an old man, you'll want to train legs now.

The following workouts cover a broad range of approaches to leg training, with at least one guaranteed to meet your requirements. Whether it's the ego boost from heavy squats, the challenge of suspension training, or fear of a lightbulb body (picture it) that motivates you to train your legs, we've got you covered.

THE BEST FULL-GYM LEG WORKOUT

WORKOUT #58   BY C.J. MURPHY, M.F.S.

If you're wondering why your legs haven't grown, ask yourself another question: "How much do I squat?" If the answer isn't at least one and a half times your body weight, you better step under the bar and get after it. Improving your squat will go further toward building big, strong legs than any other exercise, and the workout at right does it with only three exercises.

HOW IT WORKS Most people get stuck coming "out of the hole" on a squat–rising up from the bottom position. They start to pitch forward and their hips rise too fast, resulting in bad form that can cause injury or even a missed lift. Pausing at the bottom will get you comfortable with the toughest point in the range of motion. Two other exercises also help with this problem–the lunge and single-leg back extension. Working your quads and hamstrings unilaterally enhances stability and strengthens your core, so you can squat big weights solidly.

DIRECTIONS Complete all sets for one exercise before going on to the next.

1 PAUSE SQUAT

SETS: 4 REPS: 12, 10, 8, 6 REST: 120 SEC.

Set up in a squat rack or cage. Grasp the bar as far apart as is comfortable and step under it. Squeeze your shoulder blades together and nudge the bar out of the rack. Step back and stand with your feet shoulder width and your toes turned out slightly. Take a deep breath and bend your hips back, then bend your knees to lower your body as far as you can without losing the arch in your lower back. Push your knees out as you descend. Hold the bottom position for two seconds, then extend your hips to come back up, continuing to push your knees outward.

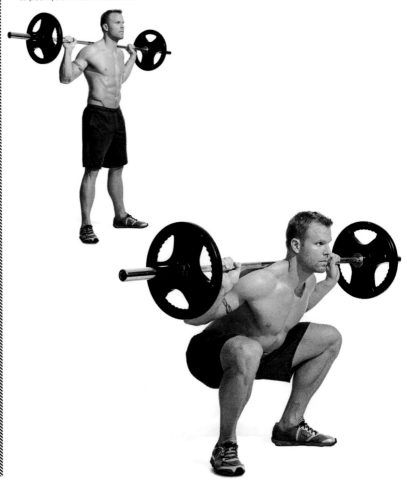

2 WALKING LUNGE

SETS: 3 REPS: 16-20 REST: 60 SEC.

Stand with your feet hip width, holding a dumbbell in each hand. Step forward with one leg and lower your body until your rear knee nearly touches the floor and your front thigh is parallel to the floor. Step forward with your rear leg to perform the next rep.

3 SINGLE-LEG BACK EXTENSION

SETS: 2 REPS: 12-15 (EACH LEG) REST: 60 SEC.

Lock one leg into a back extension bench and cross your hands in front of your chest, or if possible, hold a weight plate against the back of your head. Allow your torso to bend forward so that your hips are bent almost 90 degrees, but do not lose the arch in your lower back. Extend your hips so that your body forms a straight line.

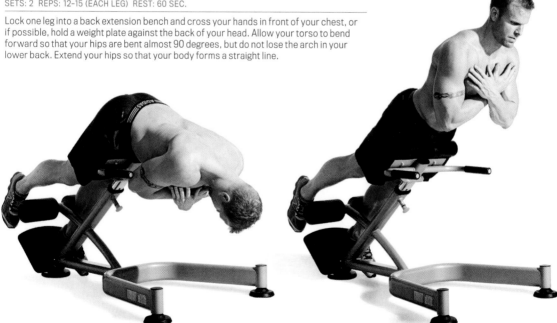

THE BEST DUMBBELL-ONLY LEG WORKOUT

WORKOUT #59   BY ZACH EVEN-ESH

Nowhere does the global threat of overpopulation seem more apparent than at the gym after five o'clock. When you can't get to the squat rack or leg press machine, this workout is the answer, and it requires only a single pair of dumbbells and a step from the aerobics studio. (If you train at home, a chair or bench will work as well.)

HOW IT WORKS The circuit we designed allows you to stay put. Grab one pair of dumbbells and a little floor space and you won't have to move until the workout is done. No matter what the traffic flow is around you, you'll be able to get through your training without competing for equipment or space.

The dumbbell stepup targets the glutes and hamstrings; the reverse lunge works the quads; and the squat, of course, hits all three. Combine these moves into a circuit done with little rest, and you'll be in and out of the gym while everyone else is still waiting for the bench.

DIRECTIONS Perform the exercises as a circuit, completing one set of each in sequence without rest. Afterward, rest 90 seconds, then repeat the circuit once more.

1 DUMBBELL STEPUP

SETS: 2 REPS: 5 (EACH SIDE) REST: 0 SEC.

Stand behind an aerobics step or other elevated surface that will put your thigh at parallel to the floor when you place your foot onto it. Hold a dumbbell in each hand and step up onto the bench, leaving your trailing leg hanging off. Step back down but leave your lead leg on the box to begin the next rep. Complete all the reps on that side and then switch. That's one set.

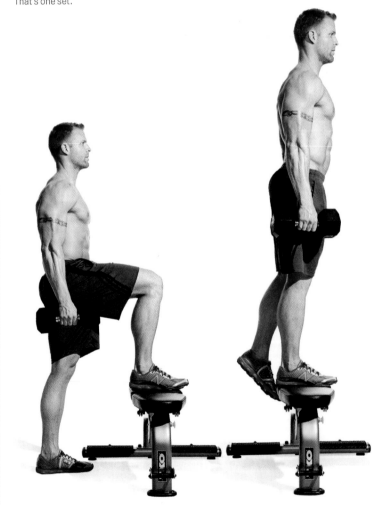

2 REVERSE LUNGE

SETS: 2 REPS: 5 (EACH SIDE)
REST: 0 SEC.

Stand with the dumbbells still in your hands and step back with your right foot. Lower your body until your front thigh is parallel to the floor and your rear knee nearly touches the floor. Keep your torso upright. Step forward to return to the starting position. Complete all reps on one leg, then switch legs. That's one set.

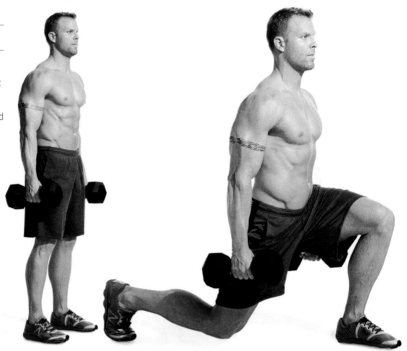

3 DUMBBELL SQUAT

SETS: 2 REPS: 10 REST: 90 SEC.

Hold the weights at shoulder level and stand with feet shoulder width and toes turned slightly out. Squat down as low as you can without losing the arch in your lower back.

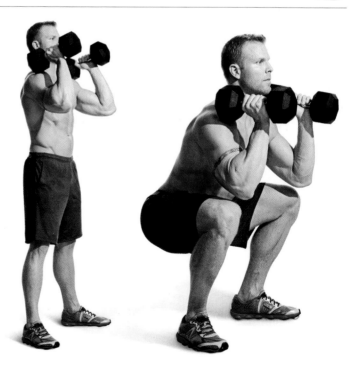

THE BEST BARBELL-ONLY LEG WORKOUT

WORKOUT #60   BY JOHN ROMANIELLO

The beauty of having only a barbell to train legs with is that you can still do squats. And even if squats were all you could do with it, you wouldn't need any other leg exercises for a long time. But the barbell is more versatile than most give it credit for—we can even show you how to work your calves with it—and when combined with some explosive bodyweight exercises, you've got a workout that's as good as practically any you'd get in a big-box gym.

HOW IT WORKS The workout is built on circuits that alternate a heavy exercise with an explosive one. The heavy lift recruits a lot of muscle fibers, and the explosive one done immediately after allows for even better muscle activation on the next heavy set. In just a few sets and a few minutes, you can stimulate as many muscle fibers as you normally would during much longer leg workouts. In addition, the combination of strength and power you'll build will help improve sprinting speed and jump height.

DIRECTIONS The workout consists of two circuits. Complete Circuit 1 as directed and then repeat once more. Then move on to Circuit 2 (which you'll perform only once).

▼ CIRCUIT 1

Immediately after your second set of the squat, perform the jump squat.

1 SQUAT

SETS: 2 REPS: 5 REST: 60 SEC. (AFTER THE FIRST SET ONLY)

Set up in a squat rack or cage. Grasp the bar as far apart as is comfortable and step under it. Squeeze your shoulder blades together and nudge the bar out of the rack. Step back and stand with your feet shoulder width and your toes turned slightly outward. Take a deep breath and then bend your hips and knees to lower your body as far as you can without losing the arch in your lower back. Push your knees outward as you descend. Extend your hips to come back up, continuing to push your knees outward.

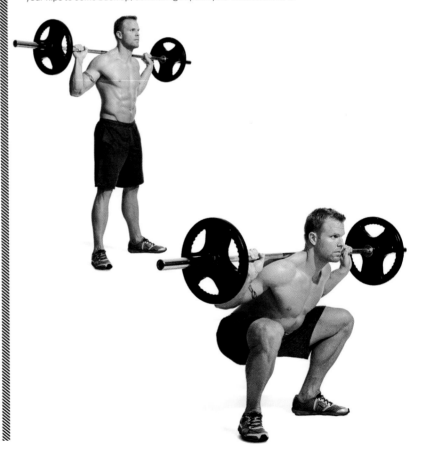

2 JUMP SQUAT

SETS: 1 REPS: AS MANY AS POSSIBLE IN 60 SEC. REST: 60 SEC.

Stand with feet shoulder width apart and squat down until your thighs are about parallel to the floor but no deeper. Jump as high as you can. Land with soft knees and begin the next rep.

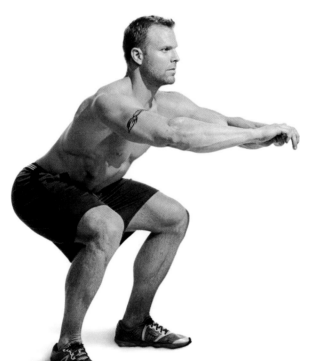
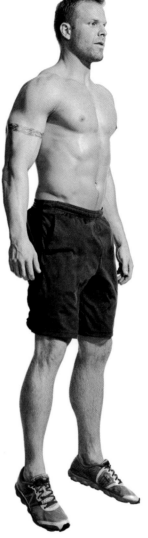

3 SQUAT

SETS: 1 REPS: 5 REST: 0 SEC.

4 JUMP SQUAT

SETS: 1 REPS: AS MANY AS POSSIBLE IN 45 SECONDS
REST: 90 SEC.

▼ CIRCUIT 2

Immediately after your second set of the barbell calf raise, perform the body-weight calf raise.

1 BARBELL CALF RAISE

SETS: 3 REPS: 6 REST: 30 SEC. (DO NOT REST AFTER THE SECOND SET)

Place a block, step, or weight plate on the floor. Grasp a barbell and hold it on the backs of your shoulders, as in a squat. Place your toes on the block so your calves are stretched, but make sure you can maintain balance. Raise your heels to come up onto the balls of your feet.

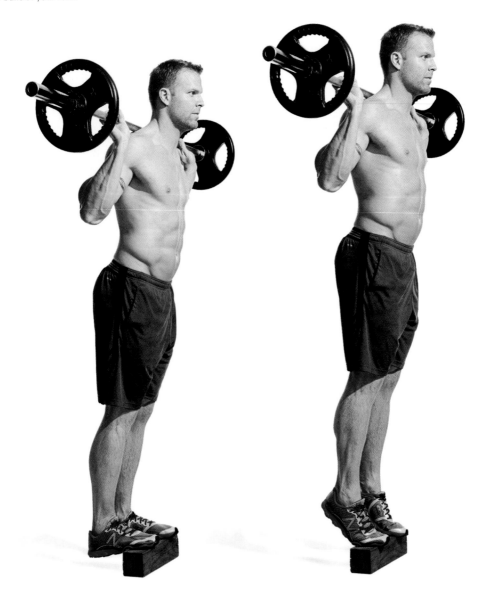

2 BODY-WEIGHT CALF RAISE

SETS: 1 REPS: AS MANY AS POSSIBLE IN 90 SEC. REST: 60 SEC.

Stand with your toes on the block and hold onto something sturdy for support. Raise your heels to come up on the balls of your feet, and then lower your heels until you feel a stretch in your calves.

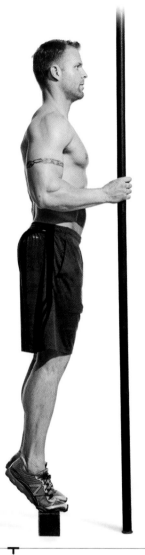 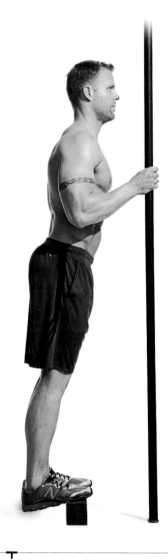

3 BARBELL CALF RAISE

SETS: 1 REPS: 6 REST: 0 SEC.

4 BODY-WEIGHT CALF RAISE

SETS: 1 REPS: AS MANY AS POSSIBLE IN 30 SEC. REST: 30 SEC.

5 BARBELL CALF RAISE

SETS: 1 REPS: 6

THE BEST SUSPENSION-TRAINER LEG WORKOUT

WORKOUT #61   BY JASON FERRUGGIA

After a few suspension trainer workouts, there's a good chance you'll be dying to use free weights again. They're much easier. This routine will challenge your balance and have your legs burning so badly (in a good way) that you'll probably want to skip them next time around, if it weren't for the results you'll see and feel.

HOW IT WORKS The moves should look familiar to you. Leg curls and split squats are commonly done with machines and dumbbells, but a suspension trainer has you do all the stabilizing yourself, which means greater muscle activation, and greater intensity.

DIRECTIONS Complete all the sets for one exercise before moving on to the next.

1 SINGLE-LEG GLUTE BRIDGE

SETS: 3   REPS: 10-15 (EACH SIDE)   REST: 60 SEC.

Attach the suspension trainer to a sturdy overhead object and lengthen one handle so it's at about knee height. Lie on your back on the floor and place the heel of your left foot in the foot cradle. Your left knee should be bent 90 degrees and your right leg extended on the floor. Brace your abs and contract your glutes to bridge your hips up off the floor. Come up so that your right leg is in the air and in line with your left thigh.

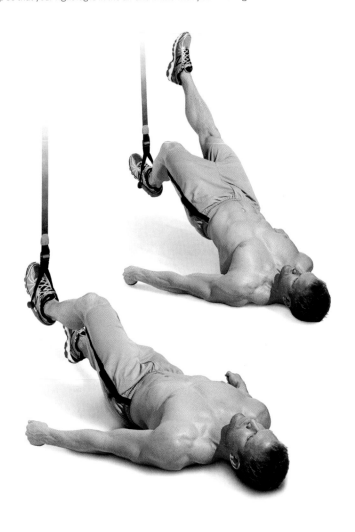

2 LEG CURL

SETS: 3   REPS: 10-15   REST: 60 SEC.

Start in the same position described at left but rest both feet in the foot cradles with legs straight. Bridge your hips up so your body forms a straight line, and then bend your knees, curling your heels toward your butt. The closer you place your hands to your sides, the more support you'll get.

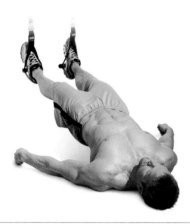
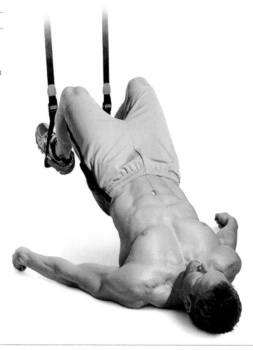

3 BULGARIAN SPLIT SQUAT

SETS: 4   REPS: 12-15 (EACH SIDE)
REST: 60 SEC.

Use the same setup as you did for the single-leg glute bridge, but stand facing away from the suspension trainer and rest your right foot in the foot cradle behind you. Make sure your left foot is lunge length in front of the trainer. Bend your hips and knee to lower your body until your rear knee nearly touches the floor. Hold on to something for support if you feel that you can't balance yourself safely.

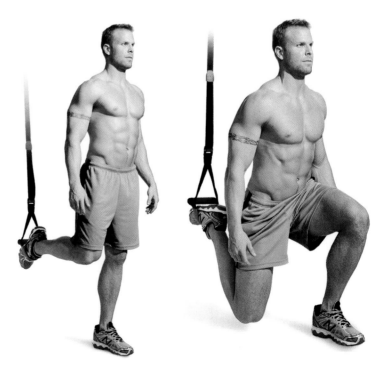

THE BEST BODY-WEIGHT LEG WORKOUT

WORKOUT #62   BY BEN BRUNO

Without weights, most trainers would tell you to do endless reps of body-weight squats and lunges for legs. Fortunately, *MF* contributor Ben Bruno isn't one of those trainers. Bruno has one of the most creative—and, perhaps, devious—minds in fitness, and he's designed a workout that may bring tears to your eyes while it adds muscle to your thighs. We can't promise you'll enjoy this routine, but we can assure you that it's not like any you've done before.

HOW IT WORKS The muscles of the legs are stubborn. They carry you around everywhere, so it takes more than body-weight squats to convince them they need to get stronger. This workout brings the pain with moves that ask the legs to work independently or without the benefit of locking the knees out (which lets them rest momentarily during a set). Correcting imbalances in your legs and keeping tension on them for prolonged periods will burn like hell, but you'll be amazed you could get such results without putting a barbell on your back, or doing the same old exercises that didn't work before.

DIRECTIONS Perform the exercise pairs (marked "A" and "B") as alternating sets. So you'll do a set of A, rest, then a set of B, rest again, and continue for all the prescribed sets.

1A JUMP SQUAT

SETS: 4 REPS: 8 REST: 60 SEC.

Stand with feet shoulder width and toes turned out. Bend your hips back and lower your body until your thighs are parallel to the floor. Immediately jump as high as you can. When you land, reset your feet and then begin the next rep.

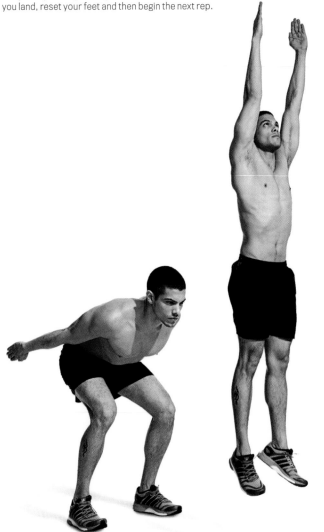

1B KNEELING HIP FLEXOR STRETCH

SETS: 3 REPS: HOLD FOR 30 SEC. (EACH SIDE) REST: 30 SEC.

Kneel down in a lunge position with your right leg in front, and rest your back knee on a towel or mat, if available. Extend your left hand above your head and let your right hand hang at your side. Contract your left glute and push your hips forward until you feel a stretch in the front of your hip. Hold for 30 seconds.

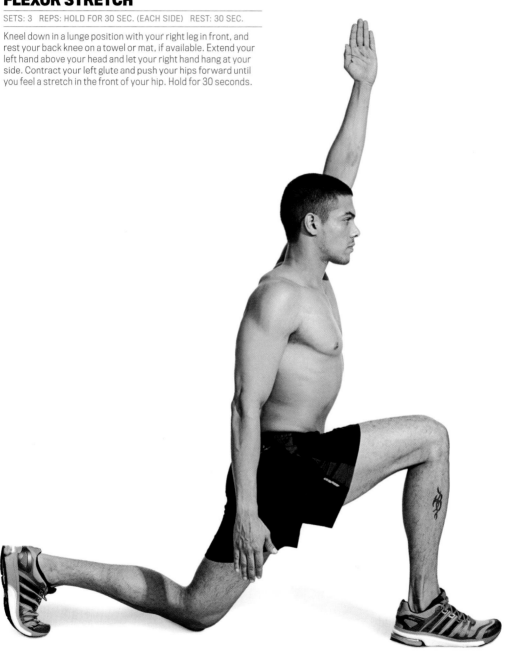

2A SKATER SQUAT

SETS: 4   REPS: 6 (EACH SIDE)
REST: 60 SEC.

Stand on your right leg and pick your
left one up off the floor. Raise both
arms in front of you to act as a coun-
terbalance. If you have light weights
or something similar to help you
keep your balance, use it. Bend your
hips and knee and lower your body
as low as you can. Come back up.

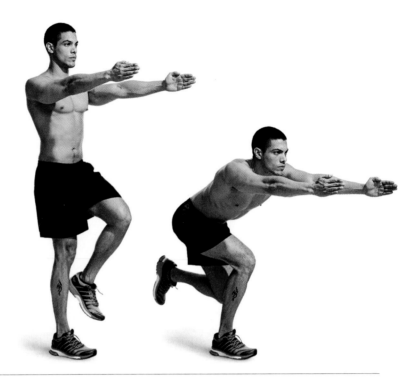

2B GLUTE-BRIDGE WALKOUT

SETS: 4   REPS: 8   REST: 60 SEC.

Lie on your back on the floor and bend your knees so your feet rest on the floor close to
your butt. Brace your abs and drive your heels into the floor to raise your hips into the air.
From there, walk your feet out in a V shape, taking small steps with your heels forward
and away from the midline of your body. Keep your hips up. Continue until your legs are
extended and then walk them back in. That's one rep.

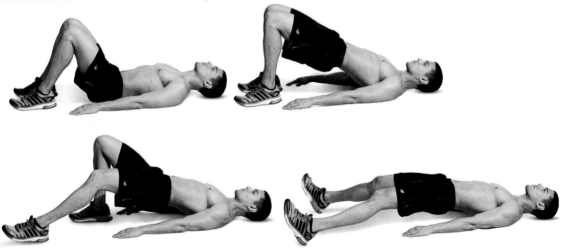

3A 1.5 WALKING LUNGE

SETS: 3   REPS: 15 (EACH SIDE)   REST: 60 SEC.

Take a big step forward with your left leg and lower your rear knee to just above the floor. Come halfway back up and then go down again. Come all the way back up, and then step forward with the right leg and repeat.

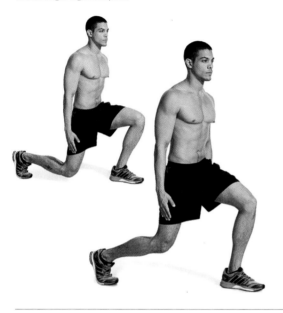

3B SINGLE-LEG GLUTE BRIDGE

SETS: 3   REPS: 12 (EACH SIDE)   REST: 60 SEC.

Lie on your back on the floor and bend both knees so that your feet rest on the floor close to your butt. Brace your abs and raise one leg up and bring the knee toward your chest. Drive the heel of the other foot into the floor. Bridge up until your body is in a straight line.

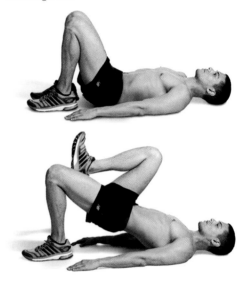

4 BULGARIAN SPLIT SQUAT ISO HOLD

SETS: 2   REPS: HOLD FOR 30-60 SEC. (EACH SIDE)   REST: 60 SEC.

Stand lunge-length in front of a bench and rest the top of your right foot on the bench behind you. Lower your body until your rear knee nearly touches the floor and your front thigh is parallel to it. Hold the position.

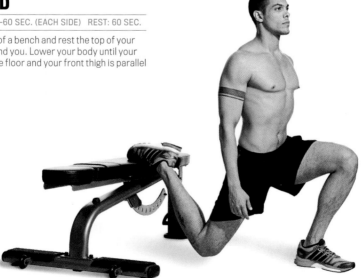

20

CALVES

You can't put them off forever. Eventually, every guy has to work his calves, even if it's only during the few months leading up to summer. We don't blame you for skipping them—even great trainers fail to program calf work into workouts because they don't contribute to overall size, strength, and athleticism like the other muscles do. But that doesn't mean they can't bring your whole physique down if they're stringy.

These routines bring the calves up fast. So if you have the patience to work them only in the late spring, that's all you'll need.

THE BEST FULL-GYM CALF WORKOUT

WORKOUT #63   BY SEAN HYSON, C.S.C.S.

Don't overlook your calves–they're key to a complete physique. Plus, while today's shorts and bathing suits do a good job hiding your thighs, your calves will always be on display during warmer months (that is, unless you refuse to wear shorts because of your calves).

This routine is grounded in progressive overload, the first rule of weight training, which means gradually increasing the reps, sets, or weights you use and thereby forcing your muscles to continually adapt by growing bigger and stronger. Tack it onto the end of any leg session.

HOW IT WORKS Instead of following strict set and rep parameters, we'll use the total-rep method. We give you a certain number of total reps to perform, no matter how many sets it takes, and then let you build on that total each time you repeat the workout.

DIRECTIONS For each move, choose a load that allows you at least 10 reps. Then perform as many sets as it takes to reach 30 total reps, resting the prescribed time between sets. The next time you do the workout, aim for 35 total reps, then 40, and so on until you reach 50. When you can perform 50 total reps in five sets or fewer, increase the weight by 20–30 pounds and start the cycle again at 30 reps.

1 STANDING CALF RAISE

SETS: AS MANY AS NEEDED   REPS: 30-50   REST: 60 SEC.

Use a standing calf raise machine, or stand on a block or step with a dumbbell in one hand while holding on to something for support with the other. Lower your heels toward the floor until you feel a stretch in your calves. Drive the balls of your feet into the foot plate and contract your calves, raising your heels as high as possible. Control the descent on each rep.

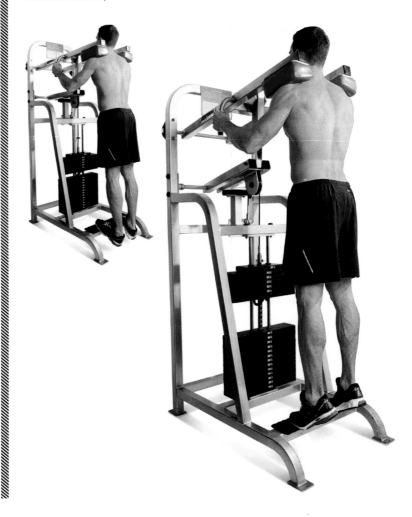

2 SEATED CALF RAISE

SETS: AS MANY AS NEEDED
REPS: 30–50   REST: 60 SEC.

Use a seated calf raise machine, or sit on a bench and rest the balls of your feet on a block or step (and hold dumbbells on your thighs for resistance). Perform a calf raise as described at left, but with hips and knees bent 90 degrees.

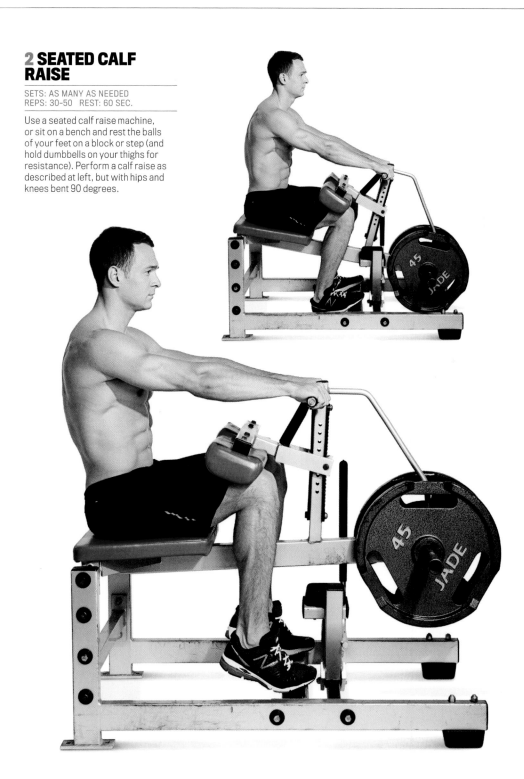

THE BEST DUMBBELL-ONLY CALF WORKOUT

WORKOUT #64   BY JIM SMITH, C.S.C.S.

Calf workouts have to be intense to be effective. Think about it: All day long you're putting stress on your calves, so they're designed for durability. If you want to make them grow you'll need to employ every trick in the book. This workout uses three of our favorites—jumps, alternating foot placement, and mobility work.

HOW IT WORKS You've probably never considered jumping jacks a calf exercise but they demand a lot from the muscles. Follow them up immediately with calf raises and you'll feel the burn fast. You'll also notice that your footing will change every time you repeat a calf raise. This is to work the muscles from all angles. Turn your toes in and you emphasize the fibers on the outer side of the calves; turn them outward and you hit the inner part harder.

Finally, you'll work on calf mobility, which you probably never have before. This is flexibility training that's specific to how your calves work in life. The more mobile your calves are, the more easily you'll be able to perform calf exercises and other lifts (such as the squat and deadlift), and the more muscle you'll be able to recruit.

DIRECTIONS Perform the paired exercises (marked "A" and "B") as supersets. So you'll do one set of A and then B before resting. Complete all the prescribed sets for the pair before moving on.

1A JUMPING JACK

SETS: 3   REPS: 10   REST: 0 SEC.

Stand with feet close together and arms at your sides. Jump and spread your legs outside shoulder width as you clap your hands overhead. Jump and return your hands and feet to the starting position.

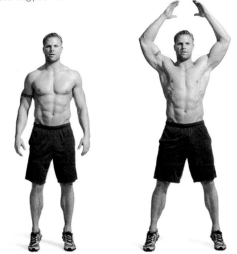

1B SEATED CALF RAISE - TOES OUT

SETS: 3   REPS: 20   REST: 30 SEC.

Use a seated calf raise machine or sit on a bench and rest the balls of your feet on a block or step (and hold dumbbells on your thighs for resistance). Your knees should be bent 90 degrees and your toes turned out about 15 degrees. Allow your heels to drift toward the floor until you feel a stretch in your calves. Now drive the balls of your feet into the platform and raise your heels as high as possible.

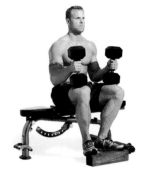
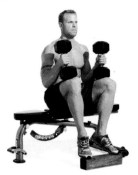

2A SEAL JUMP

SETS: 3 REPS: 10 REST: 0 SEC.

Perform jumping jacks, but extend your arms out to your sides as you jump your feet out. When you jump back, clap your hands together in front of your body.

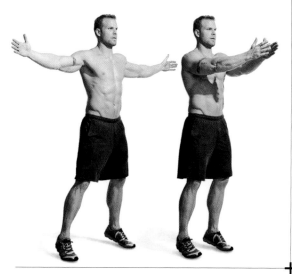

2B SEATED CALF RAISE - TOES NEUTRAL

SETS: 3 REPS: 20 REST: 30 SEC.

Perform seated calf raises as described at left, but turn your feet to point straight ahead.

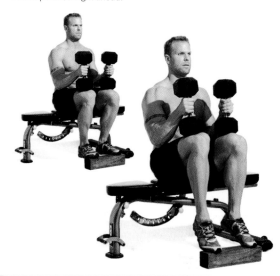

3A SEATED CALF RAISE - TOES IN

SETS: 3 REPS: 20 REST: 0 SEC.

Perform seated calf raises with your toes turned inward 15 degrees.

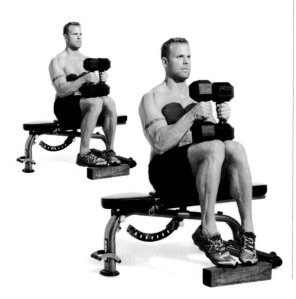

3B ANKLE MOBILIZATION

SETS: 3 REPS: 20 (EACH FOOT) REST: 30 SEC.

Place your toes on a mat or block so they're elevated above your heels. Bend one knee, pushing it forward so you feel a stretch in your calf. Draw your leg back, repeat for reps, then switch legs.

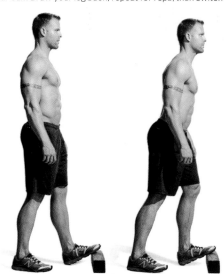

THE BEST BODY-WEIGHT CALF WORKOUT

WORKOUT #65   BY C.J. MURPHY, M.F.S.

If you're serious about building muscle, you eventually have to ask yourself how dumb you're willing to look in order to do it. Not all exercises appear cool and manly like the squat and bench press—some of them, like the ones we're prescribing here for your calves—are admittedly a little strange. But they work.

So, how dumb are you willing to look to build muscle?

HOW IT WORKS The calves need stimulation any way they can get it, and your body weight alone can be plenty, as long as you make it feel as heavy as possible. One way is to lower your body into the bottom of a squat position, putting all your weight squarely on your calves and performing calf raises from there. Another is to walk around like a ballerina on your toes. We expect you won't be doing this workout in a gym, but in the privacy of your own home, so that should save you some embarrassment. But when you see what this routine does for your calves after a few weeks, you won't feel so shy (or look so stupid).

DIRECTIONS Complete all sets for one exercise before going on to the next.

1 SINGLE-LEG CALF RAISE

SETS: 3 REPS: 20 REST: 60 SEC.

Stand on a block or step with one leg, your weight resting on the ball of your foot. Wrap your free foot around the back of the working leg. Allow your body to sink toward the floor and stretch your calf. Hold for one second and then drive the ball of your foot into the surface as you raise your heel up. Hold the top position for two seconds.

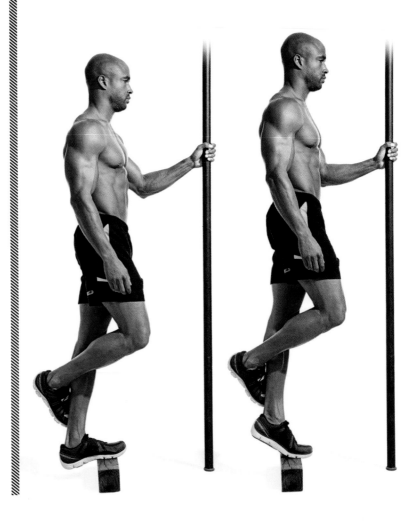

2 HOLE CALF RAISE

SETS: 4 REPS: 5 REST: 90 SEC.

Stand on an elevated surface with feet shoulder width and toes turned out. Lower yourself into the bottom position of a squat (called "the hole"). Perform a calf raise, coming up as high as you can on the balls of your feet without extending your hips or legs.

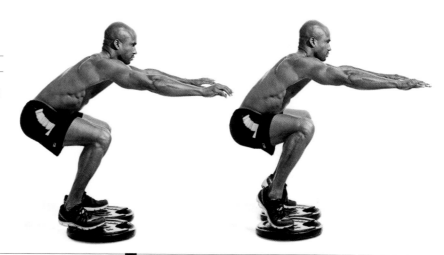

3 TIPTOE WALK

SETS: 3 REPS: WALK FOR 150–200 FEET REST: 60 SEC.

Stand on your tiptoes and walk. Do not let your heels touch the floor at any time. If you can, do these barefoot for greater muscle activation.

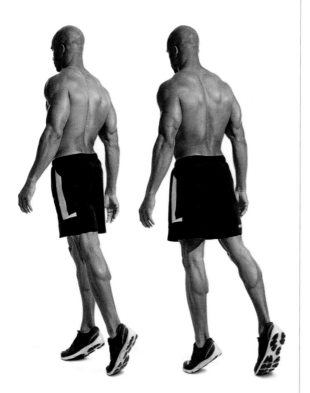

4 JUMPING CALF RAISE

SETS: 3 REPS: 5 REST: 60 SEC.

Stand tall with feet flat on the floor and jump using only your calves. Land softly, absorbing the force by dropping into a half squat; also try to land quietly.

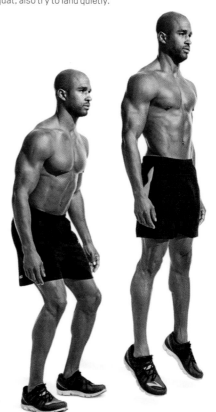

21

BUTT

We're pretty sure this is the only men's workout book that has a dedicated butt-training section, and we're proud of it. That's not to say that we expect you to train glutes with the same gusto as you do chest, but by giving more specific attention to your rear, you can build more muscle and strength while enhancing your sex appeal faster than with any other body part.

Think we've lost our minds? Give some of these workouts a go and see if all your lifts don't improve as a result. Don't be surprised if the scale also goes up (that is, if you're trying to gain muscle weight), your lower back and knees feel better, and you start getting more compliments on your ass than ever before.

THE BEST FULL-GYM BUTT WORKOUT

WORKOUT #66   BY BRET CONTRERAS

The glutes do more than just round out the back of your pants. Most guys have no idea that they're the strongest muscles in the body and the main engine behind lifting huge amounts of weight on the squat and deadlift. Your butt helps you run faster and jump higher, too, so when this workout brings up your backside, remember that it's not just for the ladies.

HOW IT WORKS The three glute exercises we've chosen may be the best known to man. The barbell hip thrust alone has been shown to activate the glute muscles more fully than any other lift—one look at it (as well as its name) and you can guess its applications.

DIRECTIONS Complete all the prescribed sets for one exercise before moving on to the next.

1 BARBELL HIP THRUST

SETS: 3   REPS: 10   REST: 60 SEC.

Rest your upper back on a bench and sit on the floor with legs extended. Roll a loaded barbell up your thighs until the bar sits on your lap (you may want to place a towel or mat on your hips or attach a pad to the bar for comfort). Brace your abs and drive your heels into the floor to extend your hips, raising them until your thighs and upper body are parallel to the floor.

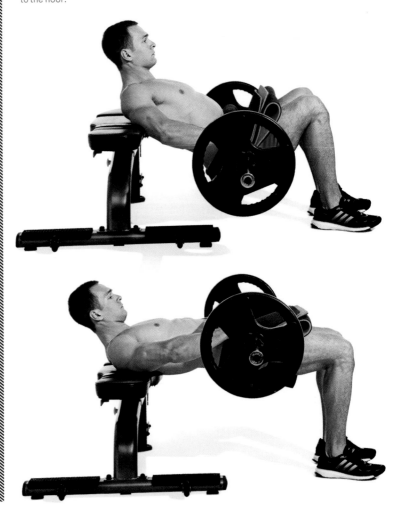

2 ONE-ARM DEFICIT REVERSE LUNGE

SETS: 3 REPS: 8 (EACH SIDE)
REST: 60 SEC.

Grasp a dumbbell in your right hand and stand on a step or block that raises you a few inches above the floor. Step back with your right foot and lower your body until your left thigh is parallel to the floor and your rear knee nearly touches the floor. Keep your torso upright. Step forward to return to the starting position.

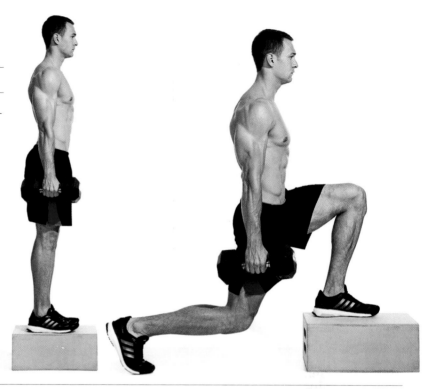

3 WALKING SINGLE-LEG ROMANIAN DEADLIFT

SETS: 3 REPS: 8 (EACH SIDE) REST: 60 SEC.

Hold a dumbbell in each hand and take a step forward with your left leg so you're in a split-stance position. Keeping your front knee slightly bent, bend at the hips as far as you can without losing the arch in your lower back. Use your glutes to straighten your torso as you step forward to begin the next rep.

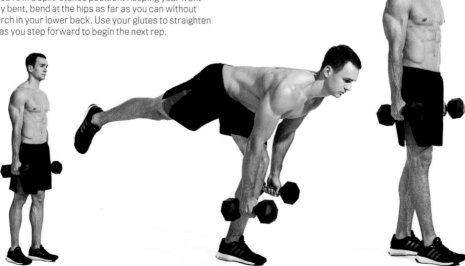

THE BEST BARBELL-ONLY BUTT WORKOUT

WORKOUT #67   BY BEN BRUNO

Your butt won't work right if your hips are tight. You won't be able to get a full contraction on squats and other exercises that work the glutes, and that robs you of gains. But when you integrate hip-opener exercises into your glute training, you can get the posterior you want while improving strength and athleticism, and warding off lower-back pain.

HOW IT WORKS The first and third exercise pairs alternate strength movements with mobility drills that open your hips. Don't skip these! They don't exactly build muscle but rather help you to build muscle indirectly by improving your ability to extend your hips. That simple motion–using the muscles in your butt to push your hips forward–is the most powerful single movement the body can perform (and the foundation for sprinting and squatting). Also, mobile hips take pressure off the lumbar spine, relieving any aches you may be dealing with back there.

DIRECTIONS Perform the exercise pairs (marked "A" and "B") as alternating sets. So you'll do a set of A, rest, then a set of B, rest again, and continue for all the prescribed sets.

1A BULGARIAN SPLIT SQUAT

SETS: 4   REPS: 5 (EACH LEG)   REST: 60 SEC.

Hold the bar on the backs of your shoulders as if to squat. Rest the top of your left foot on a bench or box behind you so that your back knee is bent 90 degrees. Bend your hips and right knee to lower your body until your rear knee nearly touches the floor.

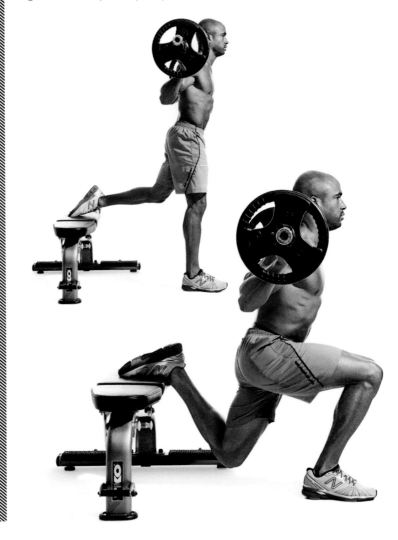

1B KNEELING HIP FLEXOR MOBILIZATION

SETS: 3   REPS: HOLD FOR 20 SEC. (EACH SIDE)   REST: 0 SEC.

Kneel down in a lunge position with your left leg in front. Rest your back knee on a towel or mat. Place your right hand on your butt and your left on your left thigh. Contract your right glute and push your hips forward until you feel a stretch in the front of your hip. Hold for a moment and then return to the starting position.

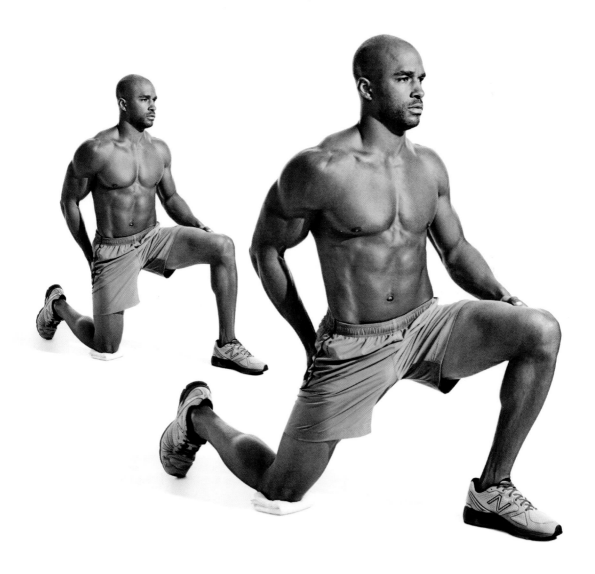

2A SUMO ROMANIAN DEADLIFT

SETS: 3 REPS: 8 REST: 60 SEC.

Stand with feet outside shoulder width and toes turned out about 15 degrees. Bend your hips back and let your knees bend as needed until you can grasp the bar at shoulder width. Your torso should be almost parallel to the floor with your chest up. Keeping your lower back in its natural arch, push your hips forward to raise the bar to lockout. To begin each subsequent rep, push your hips back and lower the bar to mid-shin level. Do not bend your knees more and make it a deadlift—the movement must come almost entirely from your hips.

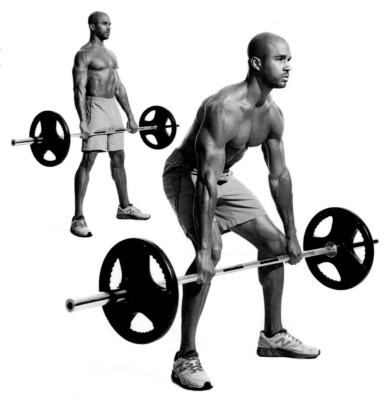

2B BARBELL GLUTE BRIDGE

SETS: 3 REPS: 10 REST: 60 SEC.

Lie on your back on the floor with legs extended. Roll the bar up your thighs until the bar sits on your lap (you may want to place a towel on your hips or attach a pad to the bar for comfort). Brace your abs and drive your heels into the floor to extend your hips, raising them until they're in line with your torso. Use the same weight you did for the Sumo RDL. Simply slide your body under the bar after you've rested, and begin the glute bridges.

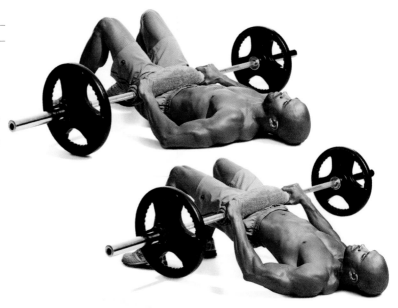

3A SQUAT

SETS: 3   REPS: 10   REST: 60 SEC.

Set up in a squat rack or cage (or, if you have only a barbell, choose a conservative weight and heave it overhead and onto the backs of your shoulders). Grasp the bar as far apart as is comfortable and step under it. Squeeze your shoulder blades together and nudge the bar out of the rack. Step back and stand with your feet shoulder width and your toes turned slightly outward. Take a deep breath and bend your hips and then knees to lower your body as far as you can without losing the arch in your lower back. Push your knees outward as you descend. Extend your hips to come back up, continuing to push your knees outward.

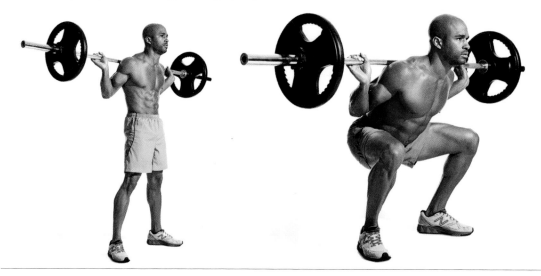

3B SIDE-LYING CLAM

SETS: 3   REPS: 10 (EACH SIDE)
REST: 0 SEC.

Lie on your side on the floor and bend your knees 90 degrees. Your knees and feet should be stacked. Place one hand on your glutes and push through your heel as you rotate your hip open, raising your knee until it points to the ceiling. The movement should look like a clamshell opening.

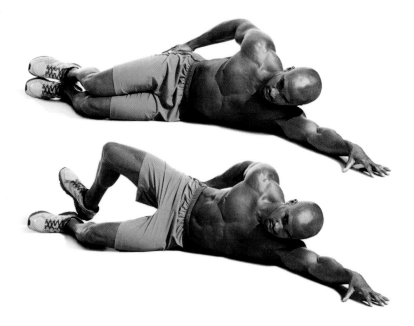

THE BEST SUSPENSION-TRAINER BUTT WORKOUT

WORKOUT #68   BY MICHAEL SCHLETTER, C.P.T.

Some exercises don't look like much, but they allow other exercises to work better. The glute bridge isn't as "sexy" as a squat, but the more proficient you get at it, the stronger your squat can be; and stronger squatting leads to a rounder, harder butt that women notice.

HOW IT WORKS Performing a single-leg glute bridge before a single-leg squat gets the glutes activated–your mind can make a stronger connection to them during training and your body is more prepared to fully recruit them when you go on to squat. Next, the glute bridges and figureheads done for high reps exhaust the muscles completely.

DIRECTIONS Perform the paired exercises (marked "A" and "B") as supersets. So you'll do one set of A and then B before resting. Complete all the prescribed sets for the pair before moving on.

1A SINGLE-LEG GLUTE BRIDGE

SETS: 4   REPS: 5 (EACH SIDE)   REST: 0 SEC.

Attach the suspension trainer to a sturdy overhead object and lengthen one handle so it's at about knee height. Lie on your back on the floor and place the heel of your left foot in the foot cradle. Bend your left knee 90 degrees and extend your right leg on the floor. Brace your abs and contract your glutes to bridge your hips off the floor while simultaneously lifting your right leg in the air until it's in line with your left thigh.

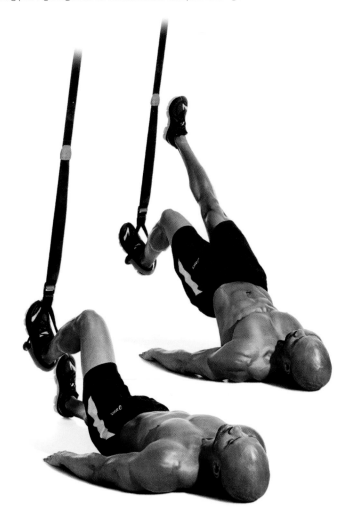

1B BULGARIAN SPLIT SQUAT

SETS: 4 REPS: 8 (EACH SIDE)
REST: 60 SEC.

Use the same setup as you did for the single-leg glute bridge, but stand facing away from the suspension trainer and rest your left foot in the foot cradle behind you. Make sure your right foot is lunge-length in front of the trainer. Bend your hips and knees to lower your body until your rear knee nearly touches the floor. Hold on to something for support if you feel you can't balance safely.

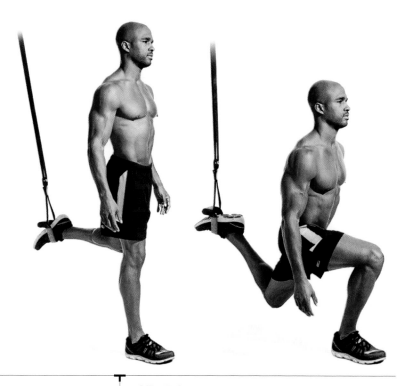

2A GLUTE-BRIDGE

SETS: 4 REPS: 12 REST: 0 SEC.

Set up as you did for the single-leg glute bridge, but rest both feet in the foot cradles. Drive through your heels to raise your hips.

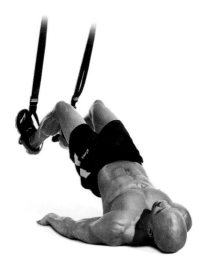

2B FIGUREHEAD

SETS: 4 REPS: AS MANY AS POSSIBLE REST: 120 SEC.

Lie on the floor facedown with your arms at your sides. Squeeze your glutes and raise your torso and legs simultaneously so only your hips touch the floor. Imagine touching your feet with your hands. Hold for a second at the top, and then return to the starting position so your shoulders touch the floor.

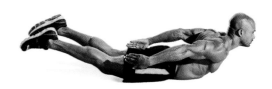

THE BEST
SWISS-BALL BUTT WORKOUT

WORKOUT #69   BY MICHAEL SCHLETTER, C.P.T.

One of the reasons a better-looking, athletic butt stands out is because of a clear division between the glutes and the hamstrings. The back of the leg comes up and then prominently curves outward to form the buttock. Strangely enough, you can actually target this specific area, and women will appreciate it if you do.

HOW IT WORKS We've added a little hamstring workout into the glute training to strengthen both muscle groups, because they work in conjunction to extend your hips, but this will also sharpen the distinction between the two where they meet on the back of the leg. Specifically, you'll fatigue your hams with hip thrusts on the ball and then finish them off with hamstring curls—your glutes will be firing as well to stabilize you.

The butterfly hip thrust provides another challenge. This one targets the gluteus medius, which is commonly underdeveloped and can lead to instability and weakness in the entire lower body. When brought up, it can also make for firmer-looking buttocks, which no one complains about.

DIRECTIONS Perform the paired exercises (marked "A" and "B") as supersets. So you'll do one set of A and then B before resting. Complete all the prescribed sets for the pair before moving on.

1A FEET-ON-BALL HIP THRUST

SETS: 3   REPS: 10   REST: 0 SEC.

Lie faceup and rest your feet on the ball. Bend your knees 90 degrees, rolling the ball toward you a bit. Brace your abs and drive through your heels to raise your hips into the air until they're in line with your torso.

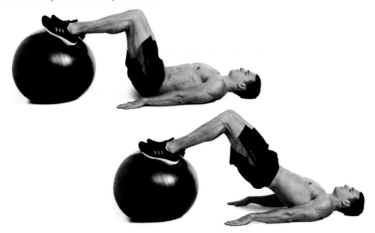

1B HAMSTRING CURL

SETS: 3   REPS: 10   REST: 90 SEC.

Brace your abs and raise your hips into the air as described above, but keep your knees straight. From there, bend your knees and roll the ball back toward you. Keep your hips elevated throughout the set.

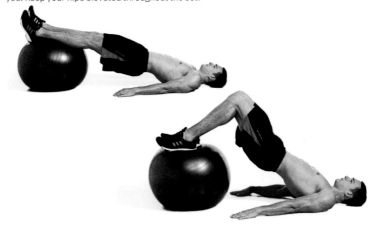

2A BUTTERFLY HIP THRUST

SETS: 4 REPS: 8 REST: 0 SEC.

Place the ball against a wall and lie back on it so your upper back is supported and your butt is in front of the ball hovering above the floor. Place the soles of your feet together and rest them on the floor in front of you. Brace your abs, push your knees out, and drive your feet into the floor to raise your hips until they're level with your torso.

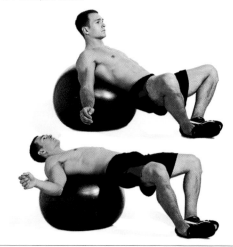

2B WALL SQUAT

SETS: 4 REPS: 10 REST: 90 SEC.

Place the ball against a wall and stand with your back against it, holding it in place. Place your feet shoulder width and turn your toes out about 15 degrees. Squat down as low as you can, rolling the ball down the wall as you descend.

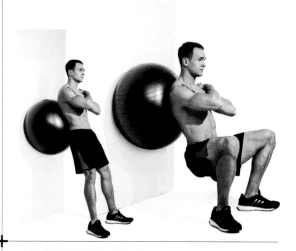

3A REVERSE BACK EXTENSION

SETS: 3 REPS: 12 REST: 0 SEC.

Lie facedown on the ball and walk your body forward so it supports your hips only, hands on the floor. Squeeze your glutes and raise your legs behind you until they're level with your torso.

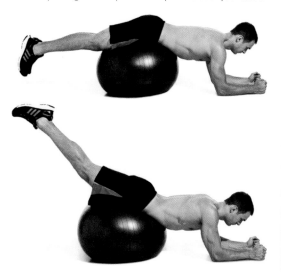

3B SINGLE-LEG GLUTE BRIDGE

SETS: 3 REPS: 5 REST: 60 SEC.

Lie faceup on the floor and place your right heel on the floor and extend the left leg. Brace your abs and contract your glutes to bridge your hips up off the floor while simultaneously raising your left leg in the air until it's in line with your right thigh.

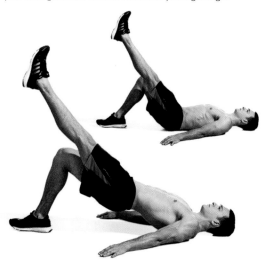

THE BEST BODY-WEIGHT BUTT WORKOUT

WORKOUT #70   BY C.J. MURPHY, M.F.S.

It's no coincidence that the best exercises for building a bigger, more defined posterior are similar to movements you make having sex. Some of them are even nicknamed "thrusts." The fact is, if you can push your hips forward powerfully, you can build a stronger backside, so this workout is (almost) as, shall we say, "sport specific" as it gets.

HOW IT WORKS You'll do hip thrusts with one and both legs and a single-leg Romanian deadlift—one of the best all-around lower-body strengtheners there is. Any similarity between better performance on this workout and in the bedroom is hardly coincidental.

DIRECTIONS Complete all the prescribed sets for one exercise before moving on to the next.

1 COOK HIP LIFT

SETS: 3   REPS: 20 (EACH SIDE)   REST: 60 SEC.

Lie faceup on the floor and pull your left knee up to your chest. Hug the shin. Bend the right leg and plant your foot on the floor close to your butt. Drive through the middle of your foot and squeeze your glutes as you bridge your hips up–they won't go high–until your hamstrings start to tense. You want to keep the tension on your glutes instead.

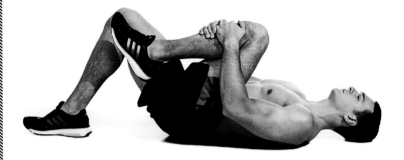

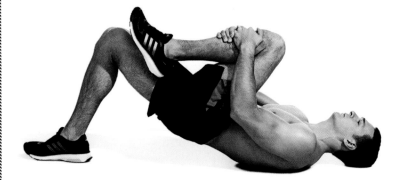

2 SINGLE-LEG ROMANIAN DEADLIFT

SETS: 4   REPS: 8   REST: 60 SEC.

Stand on your right leg and push your hips back as far as you can while reaching in front of you with both hands. Keeping your lower back arched, let your knee bend as needed while you allow your torso to move toward the floor. Go as low as you can and hold for one second. Squeeze your glutes to come back up.

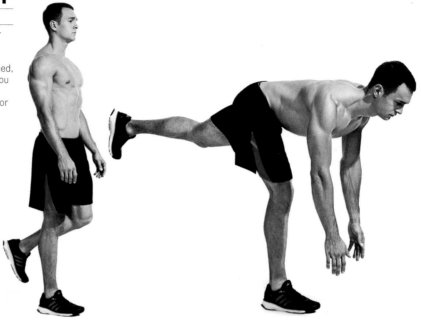

3 REVERSE TABLE-UP

SETS: 4   REPS: 8-12   REST: 60 SEC.

Sit on the floor and place your hands on the floor under your shoulders, fingers pointing in front of you. Place your feet shoulder width and squeeze your glutes. Push through your heels as you bridge your hips up. Your body should form a table, with your torso and hips parallel to the floor. Hold for two seconds.

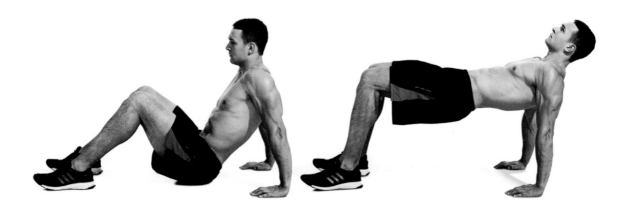

22

ABS

It's a shame for a man to die without ever seeing his abs. If this sounds like an inescapable fate, thank goodness you got to this chapter.

The ab workouts here may surprise or even shock you, as they're unconventional prescriptions for getting a six-pack to pop, which is exactly why they work so well. Combine them with the dietary plan described in chapter 1 and it won't be long before you can check "Get ripped abs" off your bucket list.

THE BEST FULL-GYM AB WORKOUT

WORKOUT #71   BY ZACH EVEN-ESH

Training your abs like a bodybuilder can lead to a good-looking six-pack. But training your abs like an athlete makes for a six-pack that can also perform. Speed, strength, and the ability to explosively move in all directions comes from the core, or rather, a core that is trained for those qualities.

HOW IT WORKS Combination moves, where you pair up different exercises to form one uber-lift, train the core to stabilize you during complex movements. This workout also pays attention to the core's many functions—flexing the spine, controlling its extension, twisting the torso side to side, and absorbing and redirecting force. The beauty of this kind of training: You can develop great abs without really thinking about it. Focus on challenging, fun, moves that remind you of your days as a high school/college athlete, and you'll recover the six-pack you haven't seen since then.

DIRECTIONS Perform the exercises as a circuit. Complete one set of each in turn without rest and then rest 60 seconds at the end. Repeat for three total circuits.

1 DIP/LEG RAISE COMBO

SETS: 3 REPS: 12 REST: 0 SEC.

Suspend yourself over the parallel bars at a dip station. Bend your knees slightly and raise your legs in front of you until they're parallel to the floor.

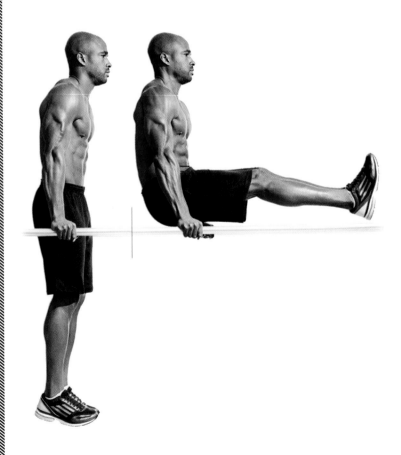

2 AB-WHEEL ROLLOUT

SETS: 3 REPS: AS MANY AS POSSIBLE REST: 0 SEC.

Kneel on the floor and hold an ab wheel beneath your shoulders. Brace your abs and roll the wheel forward until you feel you're about to lose tension in your core and your hips might sag. Roll yourself back to start. Do as many reps as you can with perfect form and end the set when you think you might break form.

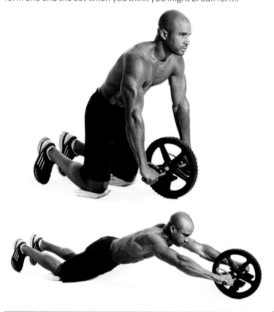

3 SITUP W/ MEDICINE-BALL THROW

SETS: 3 REPS: 10 REST: 0 SEC.

Hold a medicine ball with both hands and lie back on the floor with your knees bent and feet flat. Perform a situp and then throw the ball into a wall in front of you (or have a partner catch it and then throw it back to you). Catch the ball on the rebound and begin the next rep.

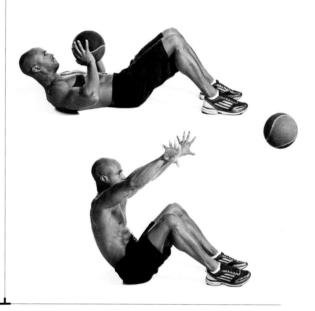

4 MEDICINE-BALL RUSSIAN TWIST

SETS: 3 REPS: 10 (EACH SIDE) REST: 60 SEC.

Sit on the floor in the top position of a situp and, holding a medicine ball with both hands, extend your arms in front of you. Explosively twist your body to one side and then twist back. Alternate sides.

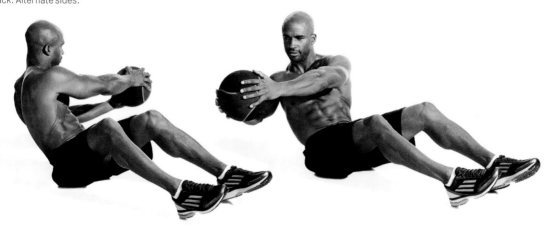

THE BEST
BARBELL-ONLY AB WORKOUT

WORKOUT #72   BY BEN BRUNO

It's possible that you have abs already but you just can't see them. There's a layer of fat over your six-pack that needs to be burned off before you can get any credit for the muscle beneath. The answer is a workout that burns fat and trains the core, and the routine at right covers both bases.

HOW IT WORKS It's true that front squats are a leg exercise and overhead presses primarily work the shoulders, but both are also major ab builders. Your core has to work hard to keep you from collapsing forward on the front squat and from bending backward on the overhead press. The suitcase deadlift makes your core brace to prevent you from bending sideways. These moves also double as great metabolism boosters. Because they're so challenging and recruit so many different muscles, they'll keep your body recovering for days, and that means you'll burn more fat at rest.

DIRECTIONS Perform the exercise pairs (marked "A" and "B") as alternating sets. So you'll do a set of A, rest, then a set of B, rest again, and continue for all the prescribed sets.

1A FRONT SQUAT

SETS: 4   REPS: 6   REST: 90 SEC.

Set a barbell on a power rack at about shoulder height (if you don't have a rack, clean it to your shoulders). Grasp the bar with hands at shoulder width and raise your elbows until your upper arms are parallel to the floor. Take the bar out of the rack and let it rest on your fingertips—as long as your elbows stay up, you'll be able to balance the bar. Step back and set your feet at shoulder width with toes turned out slightly. Squat as low as you can without losing the arch in your lower back.

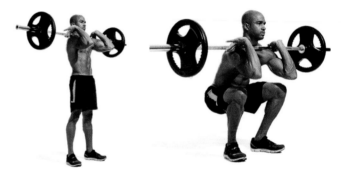

1B WALL ANKLE MOBILIZATION

SETS: 3   REPS: 10 (EACH SIDE)   REST: 0 SEC.

Stand in front of a wall with feet staggered so your right foot is forward and about two or three inches away from the wall. Place your hands on the wall for support. Keeping your right foot flat, bend your right knee and push it forward until it touches the wall. You should feel a stretch in your Achilles tendon. Bring it back and repeat for reps.

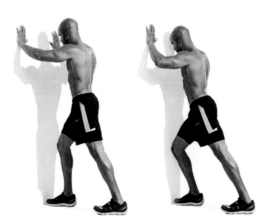

2A OVERHEAD PRESS

SETS: 4 REPS: 5 REST: 90 SEC.

Set the bar up in a squat rack or cage and grasp it just outside shoulder width. Take the bar off the rack and hold it at shoulder level with your forearms perpendicular to the floor. Squeeze the bar and brace your abs. Press the bar overhead, pushing your head forward and shrugging your traps as the bar passes your face.

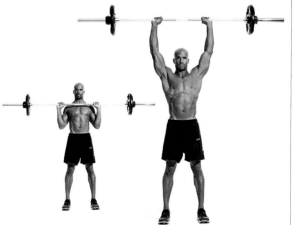

2B SUITCASE DEADLIFT

SETS: 4 REPS: 6 (EACH SIDE) REST: 90 SEC.

Load the barbell on the floor and stand to the left of it with feet hip-width apart. Bend your hips back and lower your body until you can grasp the barbell in its center with your right hand. Brace your core and, keeping your lower back in its natural arch, push through your heels to stand up and lock out your hips. Squeeze the bar hard to keep it from teetering. Focus on keeping your spine straight the entire set—do not bend laterally toward the barbell.

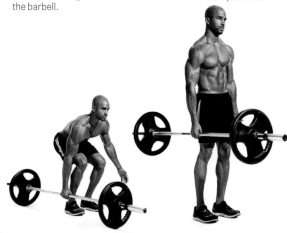

3A STRAIGHT-LEG BARBELL SITUP

SETS: 3 REPS: 8 REST: 60 SEC.

Lie on the floor holding an empty, or lightly loaded, bar over your chest as in the top of a bench press. Your legs should be extended on the floor in front of you. Perform a situp, raising your torso until it's vertical. Keep the bar over your head, so it drifts back to an overhead press position at the top of the situp.

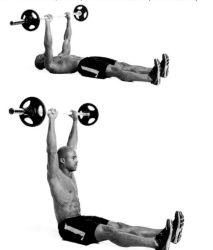

3B BARBELL ROLLOUT

SETS: 3 REPS: 8 REST: 60 SEC.

Load the bar with 10-pound plates and kneel on the floor behind it. Your shoulders should be over the bar. Brace your abs and roll the bar forward, reaching in front of you until you feel your hips are about to sag. Roll yourself back.

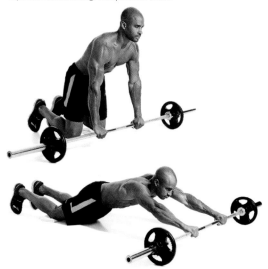

THE BEST BAND-ONLY AB WORKOUT

WORKOUT #73   BY BEN BRUNO

People tend to think of the abs like all other muscles—they cause movement. It's easy to visualize how situps, crunches, and twists work the abs because you can see them working, so these usually become a guy's go-to ab exercises. But the abs are special in that their main function is actually to resist movement, keeping the spine straight and torso locked in place regardless of what movements the arms and legs are making. When your core can prevent your torso from moving as well as it can initiate a movement, you'll have complete abdominal development.

HOW IT WORKS The exercises that follow may not look like much, but you'll feel them the next day. Your core will have to stabilize you so you keep your balance while your arms and legs are moving or in unbalanced positions.

DIRECTIONS Perform the exercises as a circuit. Complete one set of each in order and then rest 60 seconds at the end. Repeat for four total circuits.

1 PALLOF PRESS

SETS: 4   REPS: 8 (EACH SIDE)   REST: 0 SEC.

Attach a band to a sturdy object at shoulder height. Grasp the free end with one hand over the other and step away from the anchor point to put tension on the band. Turn perpendicular to the anchor point, stand with feet shoulder width, and extend your arms in front of you. The band will try to twist your body toward it—resist. Bring your hands back to your chest and then press again.

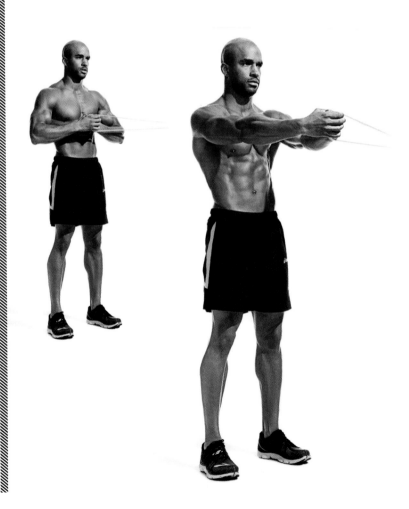

2 HALF-KNEELING CHOP

SETS: 4   REPS: 8 (EACH SIDE)   REST: 0 SEC.

Get into the bottom of a lunge position with your left leg forward and reach up over your left shoulder to grasp the band. Pull it diagonally downward across your body to the outside of your right hip.

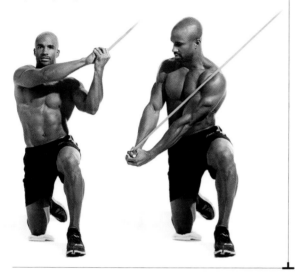

3 HALF-KNEELING LIFT

SETS: 4   REPS: 8 (EACH SIDE)   REST: 0 SEC.

Attach a band to a sturdy object low to the floor and get into the bottom of a lunge position with your right leg forward and left knee down. Grasp the band with both hands and arms extended and twist your torso to raise it over your right shoulder.

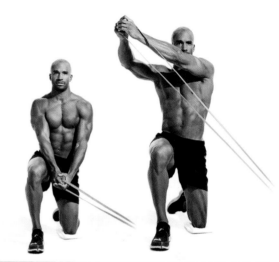

4 RESISTED REVERSE CRUNCH

SETS: 4   REPS: 12   REST: 60 SEC.

Lie on your back on the floor and wrap the band around the arches of your feet. Cross the ends of the band over each other to make an "X" and grasp the ends with opposite hands. Bend your hips and knees so that your knees are near your chest and then crunch your torso off the floor. Extend your legs while you raise your arms overhead–keep your shoulder blades off the floor. That's one rep.

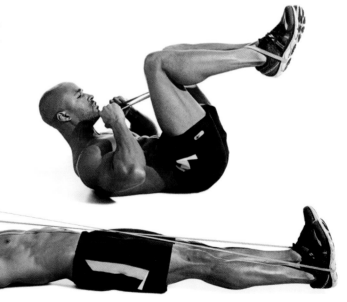

THE BEST SUSPENSION TRAINER AB WORKOUT

WORKOUT #74   BY ZACH EVEN-ESH

Suspension trainers are amazing. They can go anywhere, work every body part, and even let you run a mile without leaving the room. See what we mean on the next page.

HOW IT WORKS Exercising on a suspension trainer is like working out in an earthquake. Your core has to be engaged at all times to help you perform even the simplest movements—like tracing circles with your hands—without falling. You can even simulate a sprint on the trainer, which increases your heart rate and the amount of fat you burn while making your core hold you in place despite the movement of your legs.

DIRECTIONS Perform the exercises (marked "A" and "B") as supersets. So you'll do one set of A and then B before resting. Complete all the prescribed sets for the pair before moving on. Perform the sprinter exercise with conventional straight sets.

1A CIRCLE

SETS: 2 REPS: 10 (EACH DIRECTION) REST: 0 SEC.

Attach the suspension trainer to a sturdy overhead object and lengthen the handles so they're near the floor (you can shorten them to make the exercise easier). Get into pushup position with your hands on the handles. Keeping your body braced and straight, make circles with your hands, rotating them inward and then outward. Each complete circle is one rep.

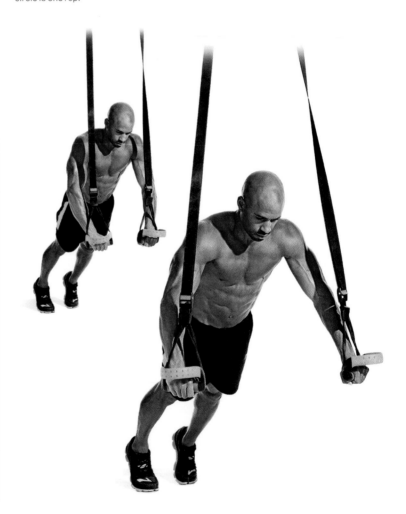

1B PIKE-UP

SETS: 2 REPS: 10 REST: 60 SEC.

From pushup position, brace your abs and bend your hips to raise your butt toward the ceiling until your hips are bent about 90 degrees. Stay on the balls of your feet the whole time.

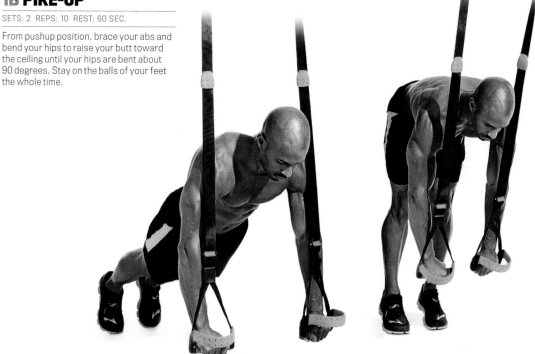

2 SPRINTER

SETS: 4 REPS: CONTINUE FOR 60 SEC., 45 SEC., 30 SEC., 15 SEC.
REST: AS LONG AS THE SET LASTS

Place your feet in the foot cradles of the trainer and get into pushup position with your hands on the floor. Drive one knee to your chest while the other leg remains extended. Now drive the opposite leg to your chest while you extend the other back. Continue so it looks like you're running in place.

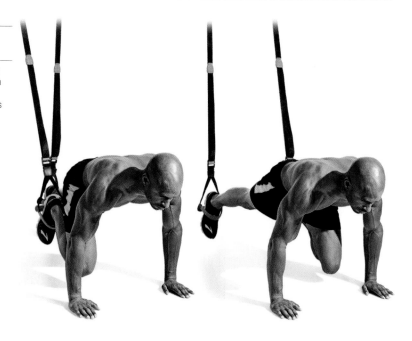

THE BEST MEDICINE-BALL AB WORKOUT

WORKOUT #75   BY MICHAEL SCHLETTER, C.P.T.

Bodybuilders of the '60s and '70s were known for taking a high-volume approach to their training. They did lots and lots of sets, aiming to completely exhaust the muscles they were working and force them to come back bigger and stronger to handle an even more relentless attack next time. We applied that mentality to classic medicine-ball training to give you a workout that's a bit more functional than what most bodybuilders do, but no less intense or effective.

HOW IT WORKS The slam is a fun move and simple to do, but don't take it lightly. Training your core to absorb and redirect force quickly has muscle-building benefits. High reps and short rests also define the workout, targeting core endurance. Training that burns doesn't exactly bring out more definition, as is widely believed in bodybuilding; but assuming your diet is helping you lose fat, your abs will pop from this kind of workout.

DIRECTIONS Perform the paired exercises (marked "A" and "B") as supersets. So you'll do one set of A and then B before resting. Complete all the prescribed sets for the pair before moving on.

1A SLAM

SETS: 3   REPS: 10   REST: 0 SEC.

Stand with feet shoulder width and hold the medicine ball with both hands. Brace your abs and reach your arms overhead and back, with elbows almost locked, until you feel a stretch in your abs. Explosively throw the ball onto the floor and catch it on the rebound.

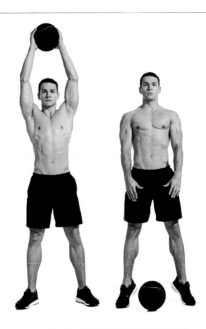

1B V-UP

SETS: 3   REPS: 20   REST: 60 SEC.

Lie on your back on the floor holding the ball with both hands behind your head. Extend you legs. Brace your abs and sit all the way up. Raise your legs simultaneously and reach for your toes with the ball. Your body should form a V shape at the top.

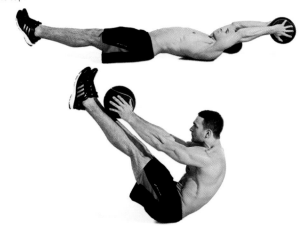

2A PUNCHER'S PUSHUP

SETS: 3 REPS: 5 (EACH SIDE) REST: 0 SEC.

Get into pushup position with your right hand on the ball. Perform a pushup and then push your right shoulder forward so you can come up higher and your left hand is suspended in the air—in line with your right hand. Return to the floor. Switch the hand on the ball and repeat.

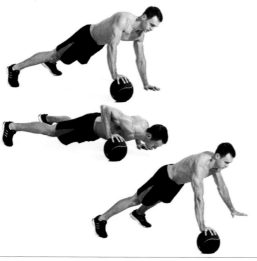

2B TOE TOUCH

SETS: 3 REPS: 15 REST: 60 SEC.

Lie on your back on the floor holding the ball with both hands and arms extended. Raise your legs straight up into the air. Crunch your torso up and reach for your toes with the ball.

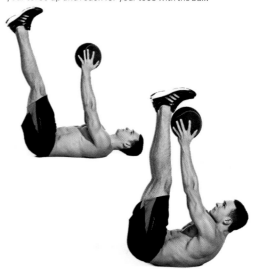

3A RUSSIAN TWIST

SETS: 3 REPS: 10 (EACH SIDE) REST: 0 SEC.

Hold the ball with both hands and sit on the floor with knees bent 90 degrees and feet flat. Extend your arms and explosively twist your body to your right. Twist to the left. That's one rep.

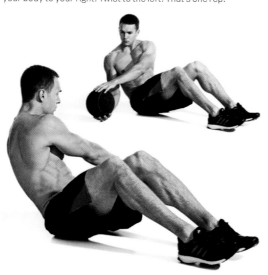

3B SIDE PLANK

SETS: 3 REPS: HOLD FOR 20 SEC. (EACH SIDE) REST: 60 SEC.

Lie on your left side resting your left forearm on the floor for support. Raise your hips up so that your body forms a straight line and brace your abs—your weight should be on your left forearm and the edge of your left foot.

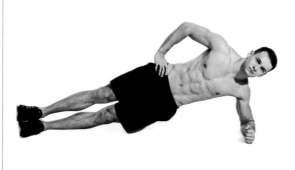

THE BEST
SWISS-BALL AB WORKOUT

WORKOUT #76   BY MICHAEL SCHLETTER, C.P.T.

The Swiss ball gives some distinct advantages over other pieces of equipment or body weight alone. It can extend the range of motion on the crunch, activating more ab muscle. It can also create instability, which forces your abs to contract harder to brace your body, and even serve as a source of resistance itself—like a weight—if you lift it. (Don't think it's heavy enough to give you a good workout? Try the V-up and pass on the next page and then tell us.)

HOW IT WORKS The ball will act as a surface, a weight, and an exercise machine in this workout, recruiting the abs, obliques, and transverse abdominis—a deep core muscle that's critical to a strong midsection and pain-free back—which most conventional ab workouts leave untouched.

DIRECTIONS Perform the paired exercises (marked "A" and "B") as supersets. So you'll do one set of A and then B before resting. Complete all the prescribed sets for the pair before moving on.

1 ROLLOUT

SETS: 3   REPS: 10   REST: 90 SEC.

Rest your forearms on the Swiss ball and extend your legs behind you. Brace your abs and roll the ball forward as you extend your arms and hips. When you feel you're about to lose tension in your abs, roll yourself back.

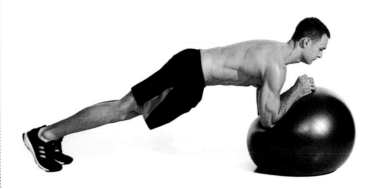

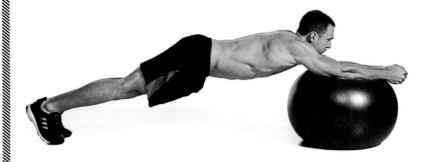

2A ELBOW CIRCLE

SETS: 3 REPS: 5 (EACH WAY) REST: 0 SEC.

Get into pushup position, resting your forearms on the ball. Brace your abs and move your elbows in a circular pattern, rolling the ball beneath them. Complete five circles in a clockwise motion and then repeat counterclockwise.

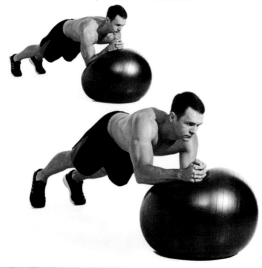

2B CRUNCH

SETS: 3 REPS: AS MANY AS POSSIBLE REST: 90 SEC.

Lie back on the ball with feet shoulder-width apart on the floor. Your lower back should be supported by the ball. Place your hands behind your ears and tuck your chin. Curl your body up off the ball until you're sitting up.

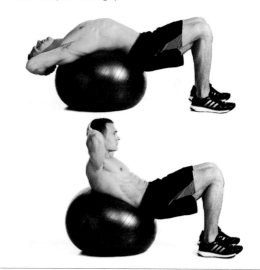

3A V-UP AND PASS

SETS: 3 REPS: 10 REST: 0 SEC.

Lie on your back on the floor and hold the ball between your ankles. Extend your arms behind your head. Sit up while raising your legs simultaneously and pass the ball from your legs to your hands. Go back down to the floor and repeat, passing the ball from your hands to your legs. Each pass is one rep.

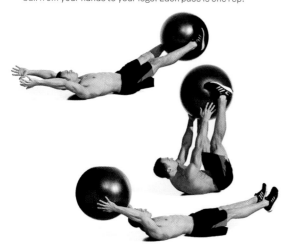

3B LEGS-ON-BALL CRUNCH

SETS: 3 REPS: AS MANY AS POSSIBLE REST: 90 SEC.

Lie back on the floor and drape your legs over the ball with hips and knees bent. Crunch your torso up to meet your legs.

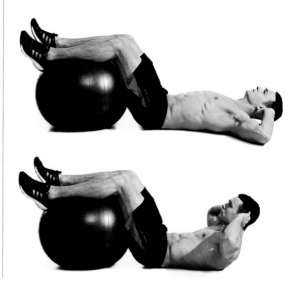

THE BEST
BODY-WEIGHT AB WORKOUT

WORKOUT #77   BY JEFF DECKER, C.P.T.

■ U.S. troops keep up with their training even when they're deployed to areas where they have nothing to work out with but the ground beneath them. If the lack of a gym membership and equipment is the excuse you've been using for avoiding workouts, let this plan—designed by a 20-year Marine—set you straight.

HOW IT WORKS Basic exercises like the leg raise and flutter kick will never die. Partly because they can be done anywhere, but mostly because they work. Unfortunately, they also burn. Working with higher reps and holding uncomfortable positions for time will condition your abs along with your heart and may toughen you up mentally, too.

DIRECTIONS Perform the exercises as a circuit, completing one set of each in sequence without rest. Afterward, rest 60 seconds, and then repeat the circuit once more.

1 LEG RAISE

SETS: 2   REPS: 10   REST: 0 SEC.

Lie on the floor and hold onto a bench or the legs of a heavy chair for support. Keep your legs straight and raise them up until they're vertical. Lower back down, but stop just short of the floor to keep tension on your abs before the next rep.

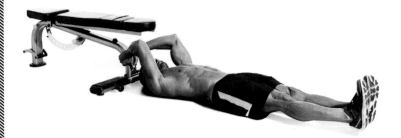

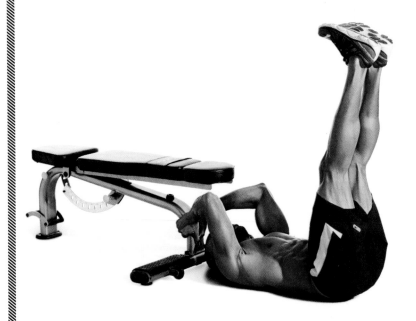

2 ARMS-HIGH PARTIAL SITUP

SETS: 2 REPS: 20 REST: 0 SEC.

Lie on your back, knees bent 90 degrees, and raise your arms straight overhead, keeping them pointing upward throughout the exercise. Sit up halfway and then return to the floor.

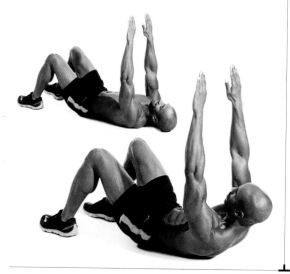

3 FLUTTER KICK

SETS: 2 REPS: 20 (EACH LEG) REST: 0 SEC.

Lie on your back with legs straight and extend your arms by your sides. Lift your heels about six inches and rapidly kick your feet up and down in a quick, scissor-like motion.

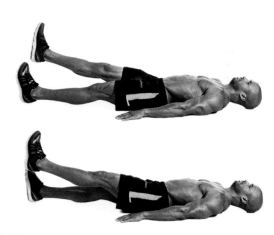

4 STAR PLANK

SETS: 2 REPS: HOLD FOR 30 SEC REST: 60 SEC.

Get into pushup position. Move your arms and feet apart as wide as possible—your body will make a star shape. Hold the position with your torso straight and abs braced for 30 seconds.

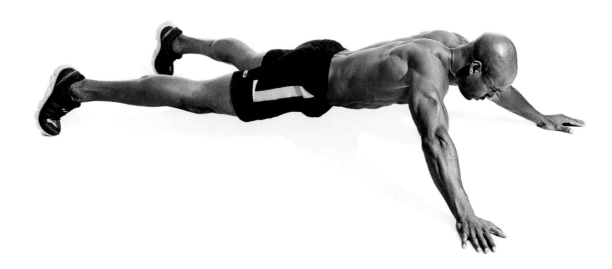

23

TRAPS

If you're a skinny guy, you probably fantasize about having big traps as much as you do big arms and pecs. Having a thick neck and traps that reach to your ears (collectively called "the yoke") is the hallmark of defensive linemen, wrestlers, bouncers, and other badasses who clearly don't work out just to look pretty. A guy who's yoked looks like he can handle business.

Getting that look isn't as hard as you might think, but you will need either a barbell or dumbbells. With them, and the following workouts, you'll never have to worry about being called a "pencil-neck geek" ever again.

THE BEST
BARBELL-ONLY TRAPS WORKOUT

WORKOUT #78   BY JASON FERRUGGIA

You've got to feel bad for would-be bodybuilders who try to isolate their traps with a dozen different exercises and still can't get them to grow—while Olympic weightlifters focus on just two lifts and their traps are up to their ears. The reason is that the snatch—one of the two exercises contested in weightlifting competition—incorporates a powerful shrugging motion that requires a lot of effort from the traps. By focusing on the snatch and its variants, you'll build traps without even thinking about it.

HOW IT WORKS Bringing up a weak body part tends to involve making the "mind-muscle connection" and working it with high reps until it burns and leaves you sore for days. But this isn't how weightlifting is done. Because the snatch is an explosive movement dependent on speed, you'll do only a few reps per set, and you won't have time to think about what the traps are doing. You'll just jump and shrug, and bigger traps will come. You'll see.

DIRECTIONS Complete all the sets for one exercise before moving on to the next.

1 SNATCH-GRIP HIGH PULL

SETS: 3   REPS: 6   REST: 60 SEC.

Stand with feet hip width, holding the bar with hands twice shoulder width. Keep your lower back arched and bend your hips back to lower the bar to just above knee height. Jump and shrug the bar so that the momentum raises it to chest level and your upper arms are parallel to the floor. Try to push your chest out as you lift the bar and contract your upper back completely.

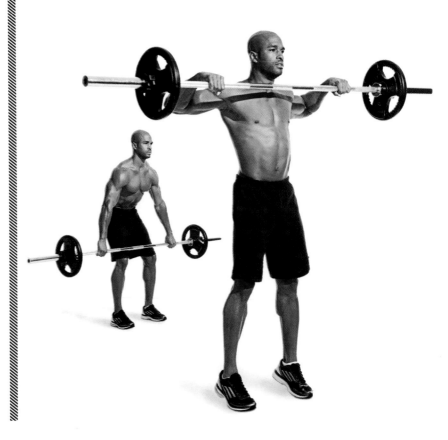

2 SNATCH-GRIP LOW PULL

SETS: 2   REPS: 6   REST: 60 SEC.

Set up as you did for the high pull, but when you jump, perform an explosive shrug and bend your elbows to pull the bar into your belly. Do not continue to lift the bar up to chest level.

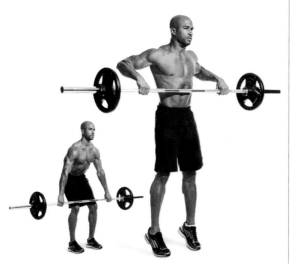

3 SNATCH-GRIP SHRUG PULL

SETS: 2   REPS: 6   REST: 60 SEC.

This is done the same as the low-pull, but keep your elbows straight and perform an explosive shrug once the bar passes your knees.

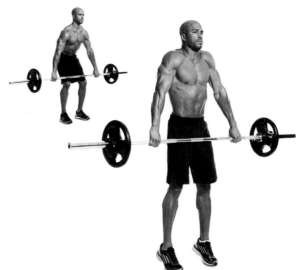

4 RACK DEADLIFT

SETS: 1   REPS: 6-8   REST: 60 SEC.

Set up the bar on some mats, boxes, or the safety rods of a power rack so that it rests just below your knees. Stand with feet hip width and, keeping your lower back in its natural arch, bend your hips back and grasp the bar just outside your knees. Pulling the bar into your body tightly, extend your hips and stand up.

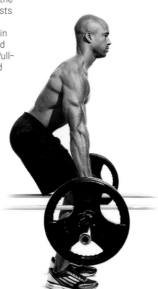
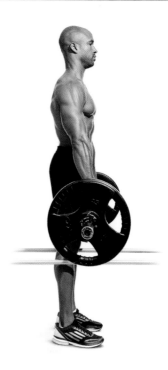

THE BEST DUMBBELL-ONLY TRAPS WORKOUT

WORKOUT #79   BY ZACH EVEN-ESH

The traps work hard even when it seems like they aren't moving. Regardless whether you're shrugging or actively pulling your shoulder blades back, if you have weights in your hands, your traps are engaged. Otherwise, your shoulders would just fall to the floor. And you don't want that.

HOW IT WORKS The workout takes advantage of the stimulation the traps get working isometrically. An exercise as simple as holding heavy dumbbells and walking trains them hard. So does a deadlift, where they stabilize your shoulder girdle while you extend your hips–but we threw in a shrug at the top for good measure.

DIRECTIONS Complete all sets for one exercise before going on to the next move.

1 FARMER'S WALK

SETS: 5   REPS: WALK FOR 150 FEET   REST: 60 SEC.

Pick up the heaviest set of dumbbells you can handle and walk. Squeeze the handles hard and walk with your chest out and shoulders back. If you don't have the space to walk in a straight line, walk in a figure-eight pattern.

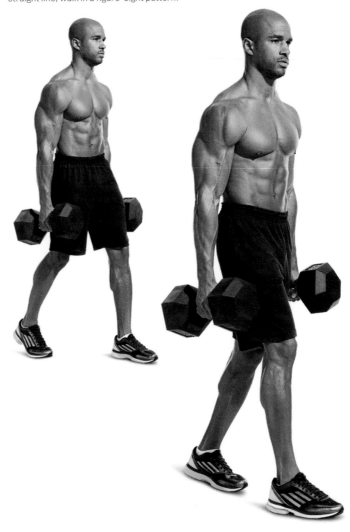

2 DEADLIFT/SHRUG COMBO

SETS: 5   REPS: 6   REST: 60 SEC.

Hold dumbbells at your sides and stand with feet shoulder width. Bend your hips back to squat down until the weights are knee level. Now explode upward and shrug hard at the top. Reset your feet before beginning the next rep.

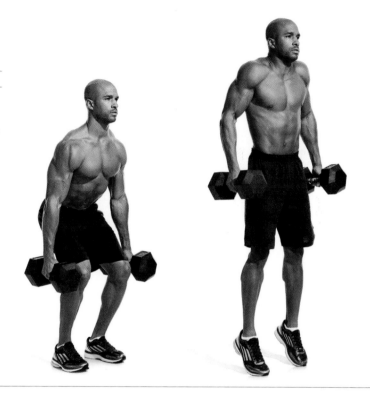

3 BENTOVER LATERAL RAISE - THUMBS UP

SETS: 3   REPS: 10-15   REST: 60 SEC.

Hold a dumbbell in each hand and, keeping your lower back in its natural arch, bend your hips back until your torso is about parallel to the floor. Allow your arms to hang. Now squeeze your shoulder blades together and raise your arms out 90 degrees, with thumbs pointing up, until your upper arms are parallel to the floor.

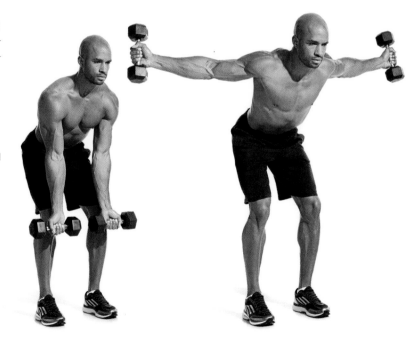

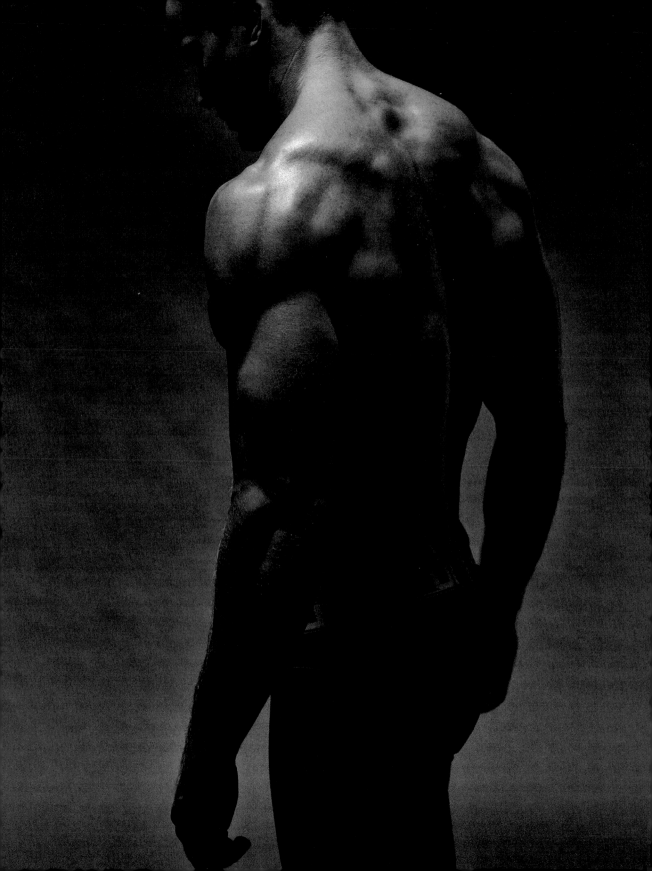

UPPER & LOWER BODY WORKOUTS

24 UPPER BODY

Most of us don't do full-body workouts anymore. Instead, we split up our body into parts that we train on different days; hence the term "split routine." Yet there exists another way—to train the entire upper body one day and the lower half another—and there are several advantages to it.

Working the whole upper body one day allows you to come back a few days later and work it again. Say you normally train your chest once every five days. You could hit it twice in three days, doubling the muscle-building stimulus simply by switching from body-part workouts to an upper-body split.

Upper-body splits are also ideal for strength building, allowing you to focus workouts around a main lift and then working all the muscles that play a part in making that lift stronger.

The upper-body workouts we've included here pair up well with the lower-body routines that follow them, something to consider if you're looking for a complete program.

THE BEST
UPPER-BODY WORKOUT [option A]

WORKOUT #80   BY C.J. MURPHY, M.F.S.

There's no magical set and rep prescription for building muscle.

Or is there?

It turns out that when you look at some of the most effective muscle- and strength-building programs, they share a common trait: The total number of reps for the main exercises usually add up to around 25. Shoot for this number and your gains will add up too.

HOW IT WORKS A moderate number of low-rep sets provide a blend of intensity and volume, which has always been associated with size and strength gains. Almost any combination will work: five sets of five, six sets of four, or eight sets of three all allow you to put some work in with big, challenging loads, and that's as much math as any meathead should have to do in the gym.

DIRECTIONS The first time you perform the workout, you'll hit 25 reps for the main lifts by completing five sets of five, as shown. If you repeat the workout, perform six sets of four reps. In the next session, do eight sets of three. Do not perform this workout more than twice a week, and allow at least three days before repeating it. On each lift that you use the 25-rep rule for, spend the first three or four sets warming up so that only the last two are done with heavy weights. For a lower-body workout to match this one, flip to the next chapter.

1 OVERHEAD PRESS

SETS: 5   REPS: 5   REST: 90 SEC.

Set the bar up in a squat rack or cage and grasp it just outside shoulder width. Take the bar off the rack and hold it at shoulder level with your forearms perpendicular to the floor. Squeeze the bar and brace your abs. Press the bar overhead, pushing your head forward and shrugging your traps as the bar passes your face.

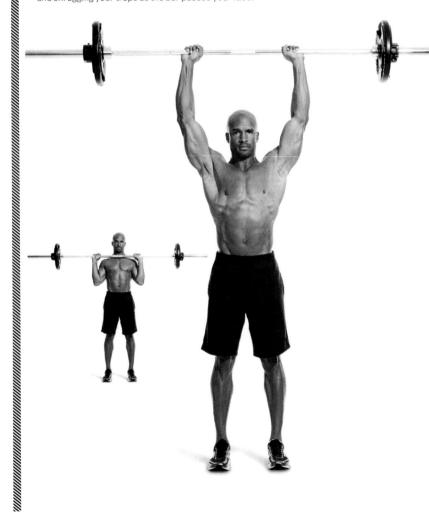

2 INCLINE BENCH PRESS

SETS: 5   REPS: 5   REST: 60-90 SEC.

Set an adjustable bench to a 30- to 45-degree angle and lie back on it. Grasp the bar just outside shoulder width, arch your back, and pull it off the rack. Lower the bar to the upper part of your chest and then drive your feet into the floor as you press it back up.

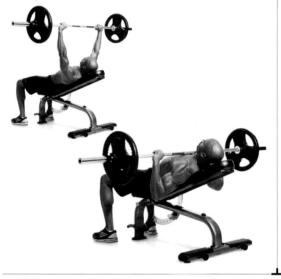

3 DIP

SETS: AS MANY AS NEEDED   REPS: 50 TOTAL   REST: 60 SEC.

Suspend yourself over parallel bars and then lower your body until your upper arms are parallel to the floor.

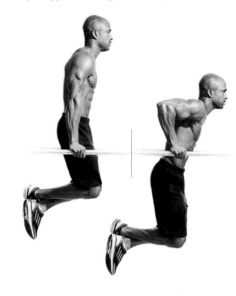

4 PULLUP

SETS: AS MANY AS NEEDED   REPS: 50 TOTAL
REST: 60 SEC.

Hang from a pullup bar with hands just outside shoulder width and palms facing away from you. Pull yourself up until your chin is over the bar.

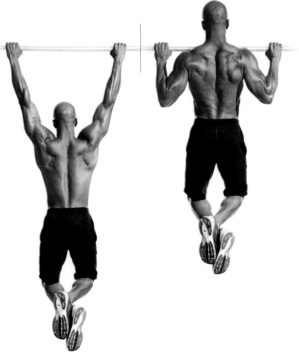

THE BEST
UPPER-BODY WORKOUT [option B]

WORKOUT #81   BY JOE DEFRANCO

Forced reps, dropsets, static holds, and various other bodybuilding techniques all have their place for building muscle. But you shouldn't place a priority on any of these techniques over simply aiming to increase your strength. If you've spent years trying to trick your muscles into new gains with fancy programs that ignored the basics, it's time you learned how to add weight to the bar.

HOW IT WORKS The max-effort method is probably the most powerful strength-building protocol available, and it's a mainstay of powerlifters and football players. It's also very simple to do: Keep adding weight to the bar until you reach the heaviest load you can handle for a given number of reps.

After you max out your bench press, you'll train the rest of the body heavy using exercises that help you to keep driving up your bench press and overall upper-body strength. As your strength increases, so will your muscle gains.

And then we'll revisit those forced reps.

DIRECTIONS Perform the paired exercises (marked "A" and "B") as supersets. So you'll do one set of A and then immediately do a set of B, rest, and repeat for the prescribed sets. For the remaining exercises, complete all sets for the move before going on to the next one.

1 BENCH PRESS

SETS: SEE BELOW   REPS: WORK UP TO A 3-REP MAX   REST: AS NEEDED

Grasp the bar just outside shoulder width and arch your back so there's space between your lower back and the bench. Pull the bar out of the rack and lower it to your sternum, tucking your elbows about 45 degrees to your sides. When the bar touches your body, drive your feet hard into the floor and press the bar back up.

Perform several warmup sets, keeping your reps to five or fewer. Gradually work up to the heaviest weight that you can perform three reps with (this should take at least five sets). Refer back to chapter 2 for instructions on how to work up appropriately. Be sure to use a spotter or perform your sets in a power rack with spotter bars in place.

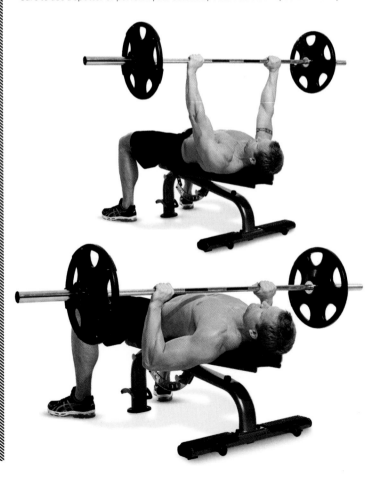

2 NEUTRAL-GRIP FLOOR PRESS

SETS: 4 REPS: 8, 8, 6, 5
REST: 180 SEC.

Grasp a dumbbell in each hand and lie back on the floor. Rest your triceps on the floor with elbows close to your sides and palms facing each other. Press the weights over your chest and then lower your triceps back to the floor, but do not rest them. Pause for a moment under tension and begin the next rep.

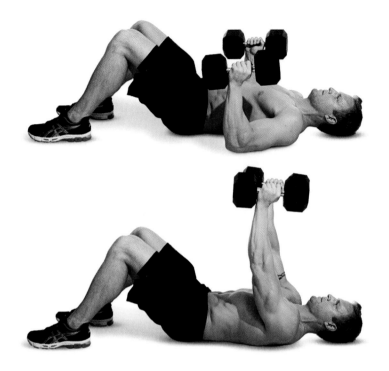

3 DUMBBELL ROW

SETS: 2 REPS: 8, 20-25 (EACH SIDE) REST: 120 SEC.

Rest your left knee and hand on a bench and grasp a dumbbell with your right hand. Let the weight hang straight down. Retract your shoulder and row the dumbbell to your side. On the second set, choose a heavy weight and "cheat" it up, performing your reps explosively and with loose form.

4A DUMBBELL LATERAL RAISE

SETS: 3   REPS: 10   REST: 0 SEC.

Hold a dumbbell in each hand and stand with palms facing each other. Raise the weights up and out 90 degrees until your arms are parallel to the floor.

4B SEATED DUMBBELL CLEAN

SETS: 3   REPS: 10   REST: 90 SEC.

Hold a dumbbell in each hand and sit on the edge of a bench. Keeping your lower back flat, lean forward. Explosively straighten your body and shrug the weights so your arms rise. Allow the momentum to flip your wrists so you catch the weights at shoulder level.

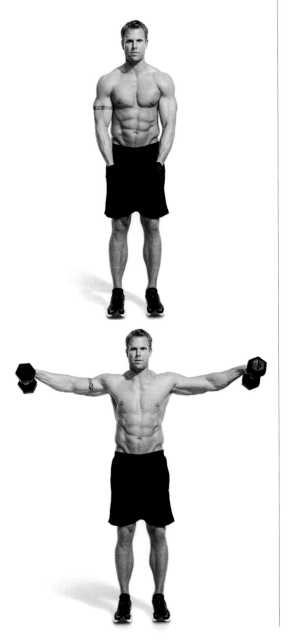

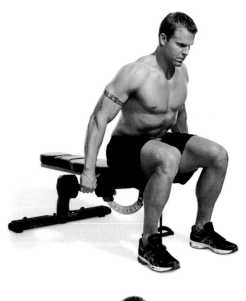

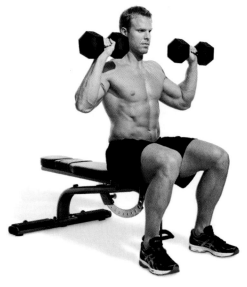

5 ZOTTMAN CURL

SETS: 3   REPS: 8   REST: 60 SEC.

Stand holding a dumbbell in each hand with palms facing your sides. Keeping your upper arms in place, curl the weights, rotating your palms to face your biceps in the top position. Turn your palms to face down, and then lower the weights slowly, as in a reverse curl. That's one rep.

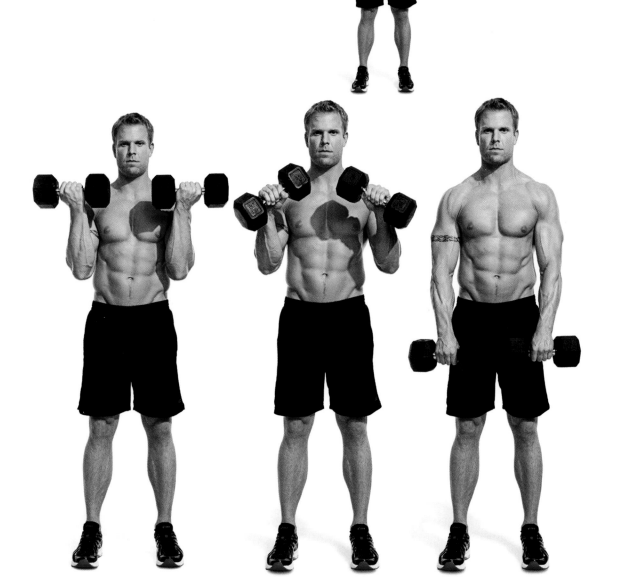

25 LOWER BODY

Because the abs and lower back are automatically involved in any kind of leg training you do it makes sense to work them on the same day you do squats or other lower-body training. This is the template for the classic lower-body split.

Combine these with the upper-body workouts on the previous pages and you can put together a six-week program for total-body muscle and strength that also adds pounds to your favorite lifts fast.

THE BEST LOWER-BODY WORKOUT [option A]

WORKOUT #82   BY C.J. MURPHY, M.F.S.

This workout employs the 25-rep method, as described previously in the Best Upper-Body Workout Option A (page 260). If you like, perform the two on consecutive days, to hit the whole body in a two-day span.

DIRECTIONS Complete all the prescribed sets for one exercise before moving on to the next.

The first time you perform the workout, you'll hit 25 reps for the squat by completing five sets of five, as shown. If you choose to repeat the workout, perform six sets of four reps. In the next session, do eight sets of three. Do not perform this workout more than twice a week, and allow at least three days before repeating.

When you use the 25-rep rule on the squat, spend the first three or four sets warming up so that only the last two are done with the heaviest weights possible.

For the remaining exercises, choose a weight that allows you 10-12 reps in your first set and perform three sets with it, getting as many reps as possible. Rest 60 seconds between sets. Set a timer before you begin. Afterward, count up all your reps and note the time. The next time you repeat the workout, try to beat that number of reps or your time. Do not add weight to an exercise until you can beat your last performance.

1 SQUAT

SETS: 5   REPS: 5   REST: 90-120 SEC.

Set up in a squat rack or cage. Grasp the bar as far apart as is comfortable and step under it. Squeeze your shoulder blades together and nudge the bar out of the rack. Step back and stand with your feet shoulder width and your toes turned slightly outward. Take a deep breath and bend your hips back, then bend your knees to lower your body as far as you can without losing the arch in your lower back. Push your knees outward as you descend. Extend your hips to come back up, continuing to push your knees outward.

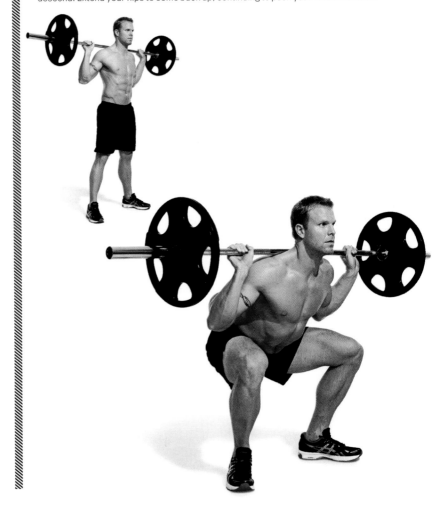

2 WALKING LUNGE

SETS: 3   REPS: SEE DIRECTIONS (EACH SIDE)   REST: 60 SEC.

Stand with your feet hip width, holding a dumbbell in each hand. Step forward with one leg and lower your body until your rear knee nearly touches the floor and your front thigh is parallel to the floor. Step forward with your rear leg to perform the next rep.

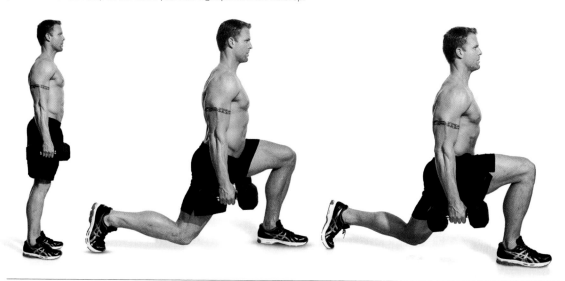

3 ROMANIAN DEADLIFT

SETS: 3   REPS: SEE DIRECTIONS   REST: 60 SEC.

Hold a barbell with a shoulder-width grip and stand with feet hip width. Bend your hips back as far as you can. Allow your knees to bend as needed while you lower the bar along your shins until you feel a stretch in your hamstrings. Keep your lower back arched throughout.

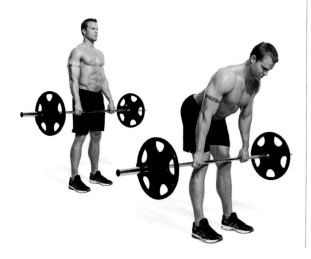

4 WEIGHTED SITUP

SETS: 3   REPS: SEE DIRECTIONS   REST: 60 SEC.

Lie on the floor holding a weight plate at your chest. Bend your knees 90 degrees with feet on the floor. Tuck your chin to your chest and sit up all the way.

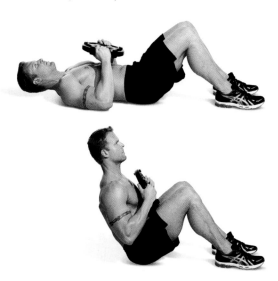

THE BEST
LOWER-BODY WORKOUT [option B]

WORKOUT #83   BY JOE DEFRANCO

■ This workout is another example of the max-effort method, as described in the Best Upper-Body Workout Option B (page 262). You can perform the two back-to-back, to train your entire body over a two-day period.

DIRECTIONS Perform the paired exercises (marked "A" and "B") as supersets. So you'll do one set of A and then immediately do a set of B, rest, and repeat for the prescribed sets. For the remaining exercises, complete all sets for the move before going on to the next one.

1 BOX SQUAT

SETS: SEE BELOW   REPS: WORK UP TO A 3-REP MAX   REST: AS NEEDED

Set a box behind you so that when you squat down on it the creases of your hips are below your knees. Now set up in a squat rack or cage. Grasp the bar as far apart as is comfortable and step under it. Squeeze your shoulder blades together and nudge the bar out of the rack. Step back and stand with your feet shoulder width and your toes turned slightly outward. Take a deep breath and bend your hips back and then bend your knees to lower your body until you're on the box. Pause for a moment but don't relax, and then extend your hips to come back up.

Perform several warmup sets, keeping your reps to five or fewer. Gradually work up to the heaviest weight that you can perform three reps with (this should take at least five sets). Refer back to chapter 2 for instructions on how to work up appropriately. Be sure to use a spotter or perform your sets in a power rack with spotter bars in place.

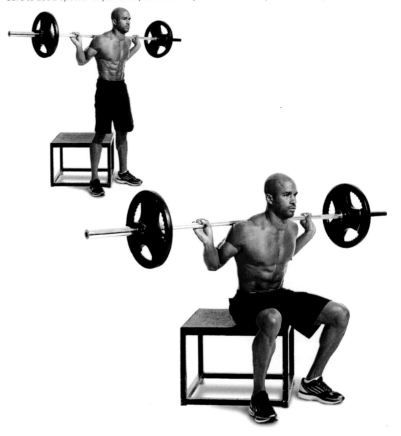

2 1½ BULGARIAN SPLIT SQUAT

SETS: 3   REPS: 8 x 1½ REPS (EACH SIDE)   REST: 180 SEC.

Stand lunge-length in front of a bench. Hold a dumbbell in each
hand and rest the top of your right foot on the bench behind
you. Lower your body until your rear knee nearly touches the
floor and your front thigh is parallel. Come back up halfway
and then lower to the floor again. Now come all the way up.
That's one "1½ rep."

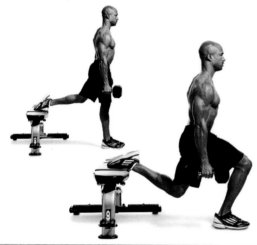

3A WEIGHTED BACK EXTENSION

SETS: 4   REPS: 12   REST: 0 SEC.

Lock your legs into a back extension bench and hold a weight
plate against the back of your head. Allow your torso to bend
forward so that your hips are bent almost 90 degrees, but do not
lose the arch in your lower back. Extend your hips so that your
body forms a straight line.

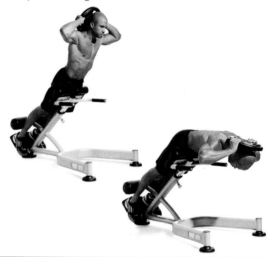

3B DUMBBELL SIDE BEND

SETS: 4   REPS: 12 (EACH SIDE)   REST: 90 SEC.

Hold a dumbbell at your side with one hand, palm facing in.
Bend your torso to that side as far as you can, allowing the
weight to pull you down. Do not let your body twist so that
you bend forward.

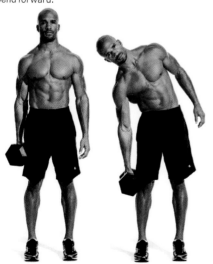

4 SPRINTER SITUP

SETS: 3   REPS: 15 (EACH SIDE)   REST: 60 SEC.

Lie on your back and extend your legs. Bend your right hip
and knee 90 degrees while you perform a situp, swinging your
left arm forward and right arm back. Repeat on the opposite
side. Perform the reps rhythmically so the motion looks like
you're sprinting.

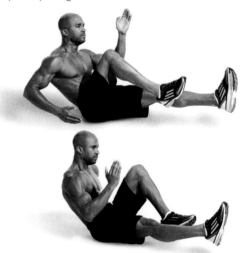

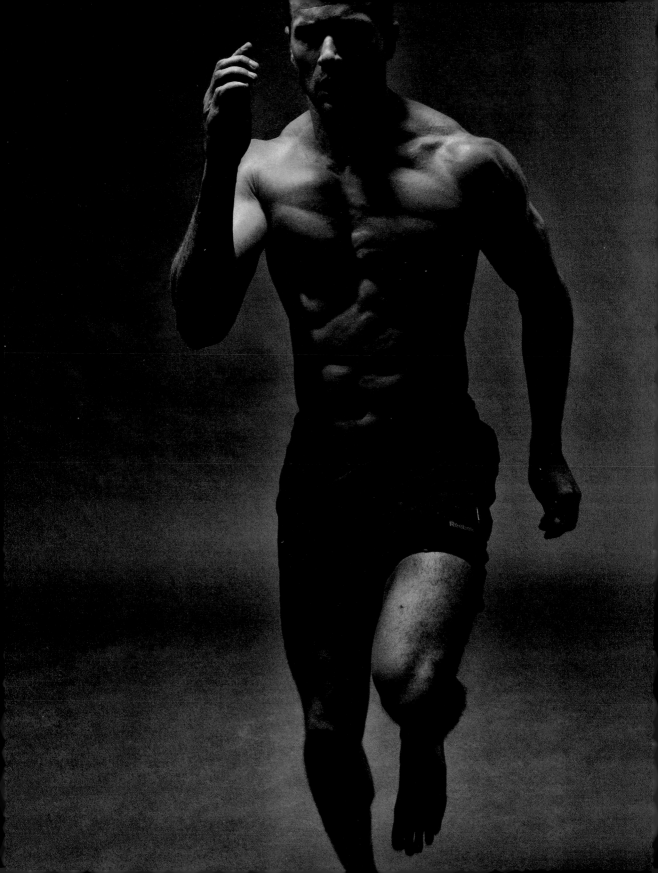

CARDIO

26 CARDIO MACHINES

Machines aren't often the best choice for building muscle, but they work just fine for getting your heart rate up and keeping it there. Choose your weapon—be it the treadmill, elliptical, rower, stationary bike, stair climber, or any combination thereof—and learn how to use it to melt off the fat.

THE BEST CARDIO-MACHINE WORKOUT

WORKOUT #84   BY JIM SMITH, C.S.C.S.

When you're bored of the treadmill, don't stop doing cardio. If you take advantage of all the cardio machines at your gym, none of them will seem like drudgery. This routine mixes equipment to keep your heart pounding and your mind focused.

HOW IT WORKS We've made a circuit of all the best cardio machines—the treadmill, elliptical, stationary bike, and rower. Spend a minute on each and gauge your intensity by how hard they feel. You'll work as hard as you ever did on any one machine before, but you won't notice it. This 30-minute workout will be over in no time.

DIRECTIONS Spend one minute on each piece of equipment and repeat for rounds. Gauge your intensity with the rating of perceived exertion (RPE)—a simple 1 to 10 scale where "1" is relaxed and "10" is all-out effort. Rest only as long as it takes to transition between stations. Specific RPEs have been set for you for each round, but the machines are interchangeable. So if you can't do the exercises in the order shown, don't worry about it. Just hit the right RPE on each machine in turn.

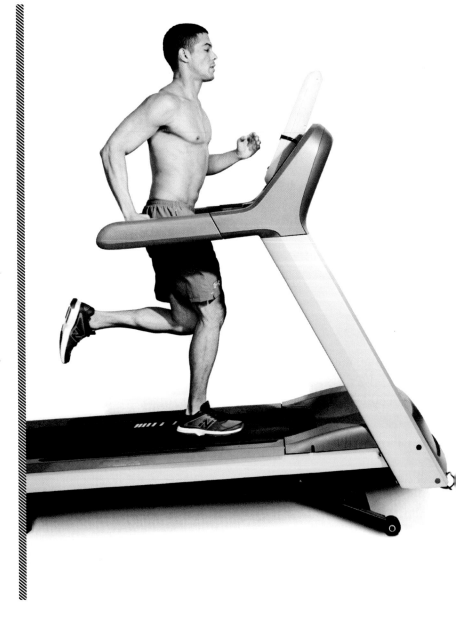

WARMUP

Jog on the treadmill at an RPE of 3 for two minutes.

ROUND 1

One minute each at an RPE of 5; rest three minutes.

ROUND 2

One minute each at an RPE of 8; rest three minutes.

ROUND 3

One minute each at an RPE of 8 for the elliptical and rower, and 10 for the bike and treadmill.

COOLDOWN

Use any one of the machines at an RPE of 3–5 for 10 minutes.

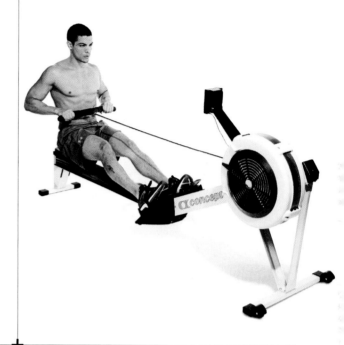

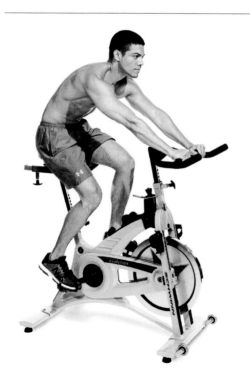

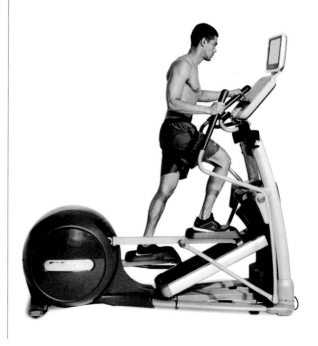

THE BEST TREADMILL WORKOUT

WORKOUT #85   BY ZACH EVEN-ESH

Some people walk and others run. Some jog while others do intervals. Both long-duration and short-burst styles of cardio strengthen the heart and burn fat, so no matter which category you prefer, you need to embrace both for maximum conditioning and fat loss. This workout blends them seamlessly.

HOW IT WORKS The workout breaks down into blocks of brisk walking, jogging, and light walking for active recovery. You'll begin your runs somewhat fatigued from the steep incline walking you do beforehand, and this will take your heart rate near its max. Before you burn out, you back off to a lighter pace to catch your breath, and then the cycle begins again.

BLOCK 1

- ▸ Set the treadmill on a 9-degree incline and walk 60 seconds.
- ▸ Decrease the incline to 3 degrees and run at the fastest speed you can maintain for 120 seconds.
- ▸ Slow down to a walk for 60 seconds.

BLOCK 2

- ▸ Increase the incline to 8 degrees and walk for 60 seconds.
- ▸ Decrease the incline to 4 degrees and run as fast as you can for 120 seconds.
- ▸ Reduce the incline to 3 degrees and walk 60 seconds.

BLOCK 3

- ▸ Raise the incline to 7 degrees and walk 60 seconds.
- ▸ Lower the incline to 5 degrees and run as fast as you can for 120 seconds.
- ▸ Reduce the incline to 3 degrees and walk 60 seconds.

BLOCK 4

- ▸ Increase the incline to 4 degrees and run four minutes.
- ▸ Walk on the 4-degree incline for five minutes.

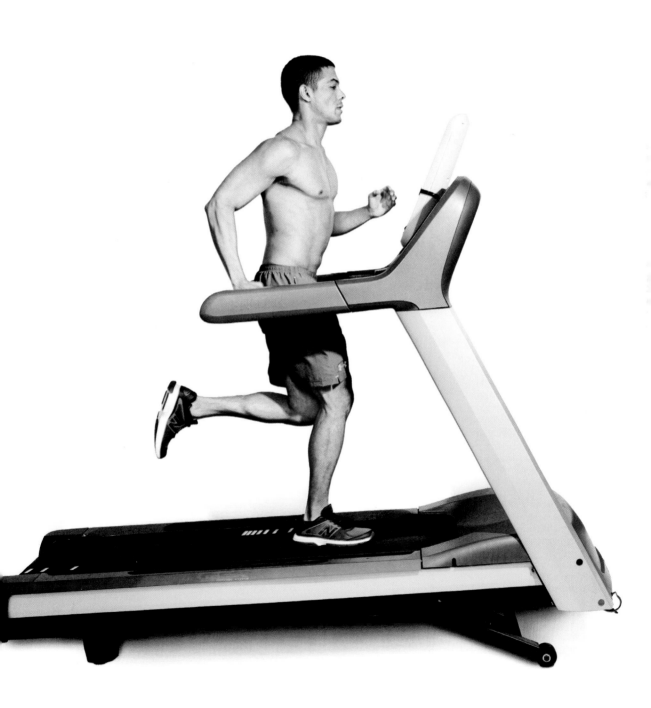

THE BEST ELLIPTICAL WORKOUT

WORKOUT #86   BY MICHAEL SCHLETTER, C.P.T.

The elliptical machine offers one of the most low-impact cardio workouts possible. This routine lasts only 25 minutes, and the only pounding you'll feel will be in your chest.

HOW IT WORKS You'll be doing intervals, gradually increasing the duration of your work interval while decreasing the length of the rest intervals. This intensifies the fat-burning effect while giving a constant stimulus to the heart and lungs.

DIRECTIONS Alternate work intervals and rest intervals on the elliptical. The pace you work at will be based on a percentage of your maximum heart rate (MHR). To estimate your MHR, subtract your age from 220. (So, a 30-year-old would have an approximate MHR of 190 beats per minute.) Your work interval (WI) will be 85% of that number, and your rest interval (RI) will be 55%.

For example, a 30-year-old man will keep his heart rate at 160 beats per minute during the work interval and then reduce his effort to around 100 beats per minute for the rest interval. Note that the rest interval does not mean complete rest, but a very easy pace. If you don't have a heart rate monitor, you can estimate your heart rate by putting your index and middle fingers to your carotid artery (to the left of your throat) and counting the beats in your pulse for six seconds. Take that number and multiply it by 10 to get your beats per minute.

WORK INTERVAL
85% OF MHR

REST INTERVAL
55% OF MHR

0:00 – 5:00	WARMUP
5:00 – 5:15	
5:15 – 6:00	
6:00 – 6:15	
6:15 – 7:00	
7:00 – 7:15	
7:15 – 8:00	
8:00 – 8:15	
8:15 – 9:00	
9:00 – 9:15	
9:15 – 10:00	
10:00 – 10:30	
10:30 – 11:15	
11:15 – 11:45	
11:45 – 12:30	
12:30 – 13:00	
13:00 – 14:30	
14:30 – 15:00	
15:00 – 16:30	
16:30 – 17:00	
17:00 – 18:30	
18:30 – 19:15	
19:15 – 20:00	
20:00 25:00	COOLDOWN

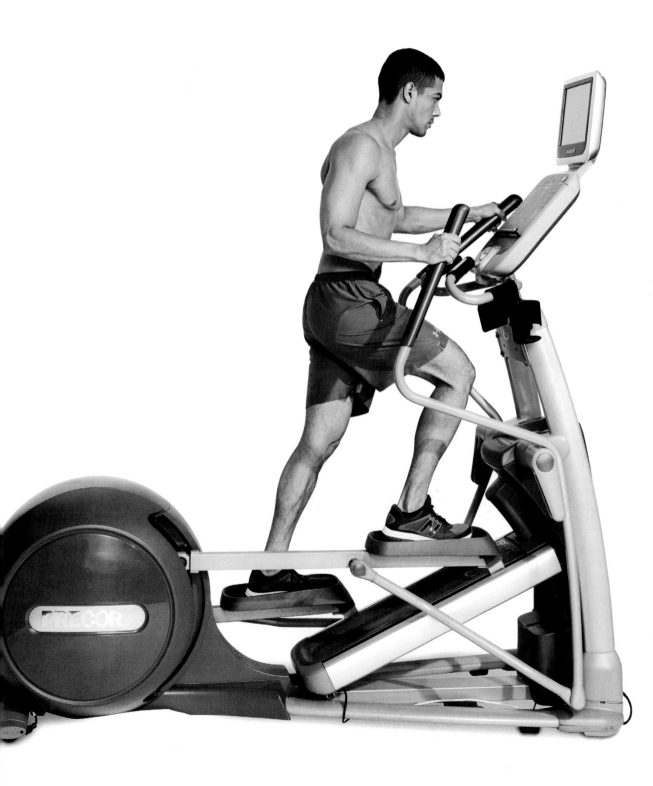

THE BEST ROWING-MACHINE WORKOUT

WORKOUT #87   BY ZACH EVEN-ESH

Unlike running or cycling, which work only your lower half, rowing machines (or ergometers) involve almost the entire upper body as well. This means you'll burn more calories—around 500 in about 30 minutes.

HOW IT WORKS The system we use here is called the ladder method. You start light to warm up, gradually increasing the intensity until you're going all out (500 meters). Then you back off just as slowly—down the ladder—until you cool down with the same intensity you warmed up at. The effect trains you to pace yourself and maintain a high output even when you're fatigued.

DIRECTIONS Sit on the rower's seat and adjust the foot height for the size of your feet. Strap your feet onto the rower's footplates—the strap should be at or above the ball of your foot. Set the drag on the machine to between three and five (this best simulates rowing on water), grasp the handle, and sit back so your torso is almost vertical. You should feel pressure on the balls of your feet and your heels should be raised slightly off the footplate. This is the "catch" position.

Drive with your legs, dropping your heels to the footplate, to push your body back and then row the handle to your sternum. Row as fast as possible for all intervals, but take twice as long to return your body back to the catch position after each row stroke. Maintain this rhythm.

PERFORM THE FOLLOWING INTERVALS:

Row 100 meters / rest 30 seconds

Row 200 meters / rest 30 seconds

Row 300 meters / rest 30 seconds

Row 400 meters / rest 30 seconds

Row 500 meters / rest 30 seconds

Row 400 meters / rest 30 seconds

Row 300 meters / rest 30 seconds

Row 200 meters / rest 30 seconds

Row 100 meters / rest 30 seconds

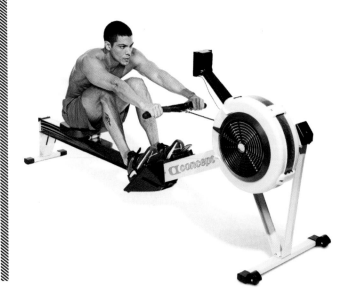

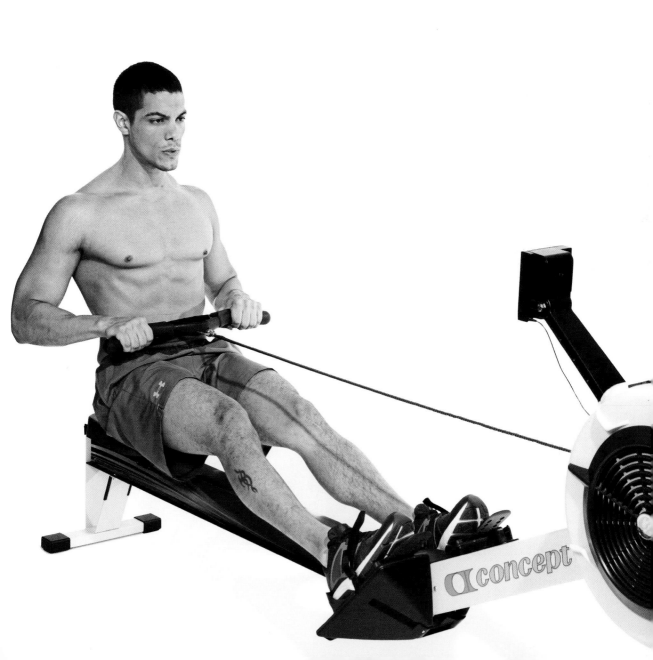

THE BEST SPIN-BIKE WORKOUT

WORKOUT #88   BY STEVE GISSELMAN

Like the elliptical machine, stationary bikes don't put much strain on the body, so you can perform hard intervals on them without fear of pounding your joints or pulling any muscles.

HOW IT WORKS Because your upper body doesn't get as involved as it is with sprinting or rowing, and there is no impact, you need to pump your legs that much harder to make up the intensity on a bike. This workout aims to provide the same metabolic output that 30 minutes of running would elicit.

DIRECTIONS Follow the prescriptions for the different intervals.

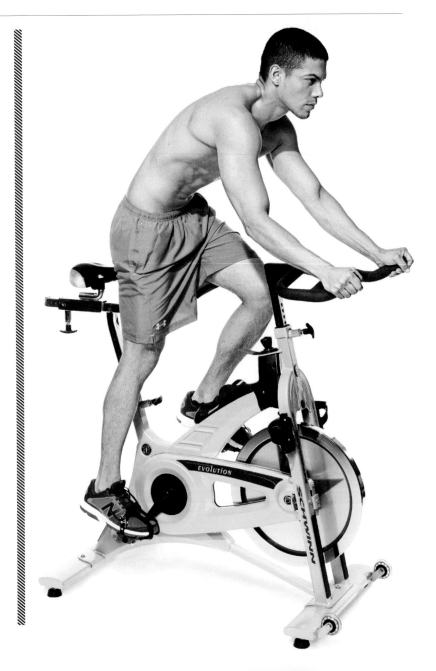

EASY SPIN
HARD SPIN
DURATION IS LISTED IN SECONDS

1			**6**			**11**			**16**	
5	10		5	60		5	15		5	10
RESISTANCE	DURATION		RESISTANCE	DURATION		RESISTANCE	DURATION		RESISTANCE	DURATION
13	10		20	60		12	15		12	10

2			**7**			**12**			**17**	
5	60		5	120		5	45		5	15
RESISTANCE	DURATION		RESISTANCE	DURATION		RESISTANCE	DURATION		RESISTANCE	DURATION
18	60		15	120		17	45		12	15

3			**8**			**13**			**18**	
5	20		5	30		5	10		5	60
RESISTANCE	DURATION		RESISTANCE	DURATION		RESISTANCE	DURATION		RESISTANCE	DURATION
14	20		15	30		12	10		15	60

4			**9**			**14**			**19**	
5	45		5	10		5	60		5	10
RESISTANCE	DURATION		RESISTANCE	DURATION		RESISTANCE	DURATION		RESISTANCE	DURATION
16	45		13	10		13	60		10	10

5			**10**			**15**			**20**	
5	10		5	75		5	120		5	120
RESISTANCE	DURATION		RESISTANCE	DURATION		RESISTANCE	DURATION		RESISTANCE	DURATION
12	10		20	75		18	120		20	120

THE BEST STAIR-CLIMBER WORKOUT

WORKOUT #89   BY MICHAEL SCHLETTER, C.P.T.

On the plus side, the stair-climber machine is easy on your joints. On the downside, it's as boring as… watching someone climb stairs. Apply intervals to your workout and you'll get it done faster and more mercifully.

HOW IT WORKS Did we say "mercifully"? That may have been an exaggeration, since these intervals are tough. Working at high-intensity paces for short durations (30 seconds) and low-intensity ones for longer (60 seconds) will help give you the benefits of both anaerobic and aerobic cardio.

DIRECTIONS Alternate between high-intensity, low-intensity, and rest intervals as shown. Base your intensity off a percentage of your maximum heart rate (MHR).

To estimate your MHR, subtract your age from 220. (So, a 30-year-old would have an approximate MHR of 190 beats per minute.) The high-intensity work sets call for a heart rate that's 85–95% of your maximum; so, a 30-year-old will keep his heart rate between 160 and 180 beats per minute during that time.

Note that the rest interval does not mean complete rest, but a very easy pace. If you don't have a heart rate monitor, you can estimate your heart rate by putting your index and middle fingers on your carotid artery (to the left of your throat) and counting the beats in your pulse for six seconds. Multiply by 10 to get beats per minute.

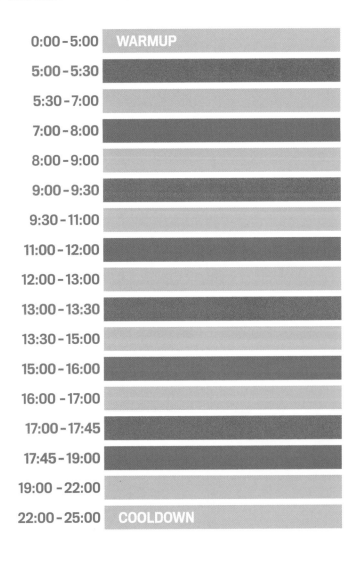

	High-intensity work sets 85–95% MHR	Low-intensity work sets 65–75% MHR	Rest intervals 50–60% MHR
0:00 – 5:00	WARMUP		
5:00 – 5:30	■		
5:30 – 7:00		■	
7:00 – 8:00	■		
8:00 – 9:00		■	
9:00 – 9:30	■		
9:30 – 11:00		■	
11:00 – 12:00	■		
12:00 – 13:00		■	
13:00 – 13:30	■		
13:30 – 15:00		■	
15:00 – 16:00	■		
16:00 – 17:00		■	
17:00 – 17:45	■		
17:45 – 19:00		■	
19:00 – 22:00			■
22:00 – 25:00	COOLDOWN		

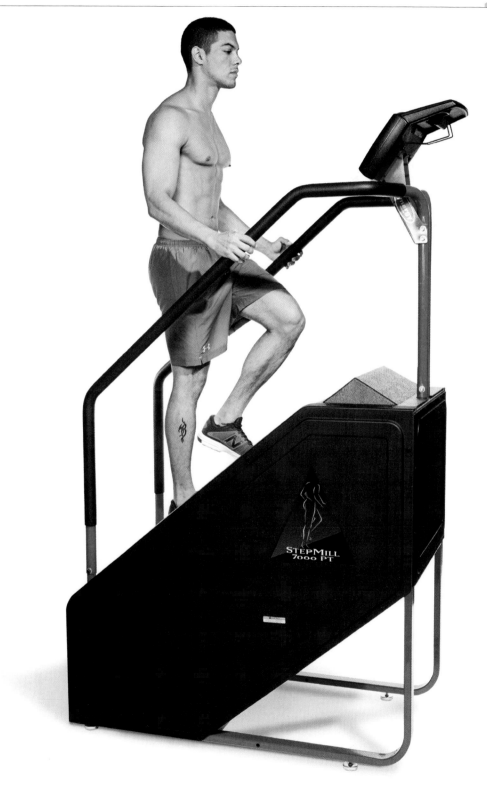

THE BEST VERSACLIMBER WORKOUT

WORKOUT #90   BY HARRY CLAY

Ask a UFC fighter what he fears most and he won't name an opponent. Getting tired in a fight–"gassing"–is more daunting than any punch, kick, or choke. That's why fighters often turn to the VersaClimber, that vertical apparatus with the handles and pedals you see making its way into the cardio aisles in gyms everywhere. Simulating a steep hill run or even mountain climbing, the Versa-Climber is gaining a reputation for providing conditioning workouts that are even scarier than fighters with nicknames like the "Axe Murderer" and "Skyscraper." But if you can face your fear, it can get you into fighting shape fast.

HOW IT WORKS Rather than assign you a specific time to work for, we're giving you certain elevations to hit (in feet). Climb to that level as fast as you can and then rest. As we've done in other pyramid-style workouts, you'll build up your distance gradually and then back it off, ensuring that your heart rate stays high and your lungs learn to make the most of the oxygen you can give them.

DIRECTIONS Strap your feet onto the pedals and bring them to the same, even height. Set the handgrips at shoulder height with medium-high tension. Begin taking shallow steps–two to four inches high–working at a 40-feet-per-minute speed. Continue for five minutes to warm up. Then perform the following intervals.

1 100-FOOT CLIMB
Climb 100 feet as fast as you can, then back off to an easy pace for 20 seconds.

2 200-FOOT CLIMB
Climb 200 feet as fast as you can, then back off to an easy pace for 30 seconds.

3 400-FOOT CLIMB
Climb 400 feet as fast as you can, then back off to an easy pace for 40 seconds.

4 200-FOOT CLIMB
Repeat as described above.

5 100-FOOT CLIMB
Repeat as described above.

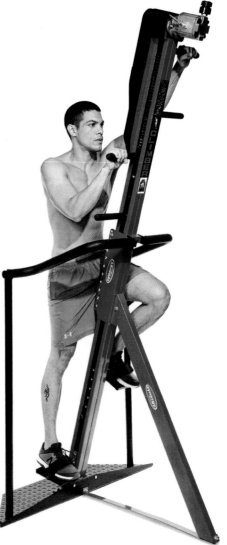

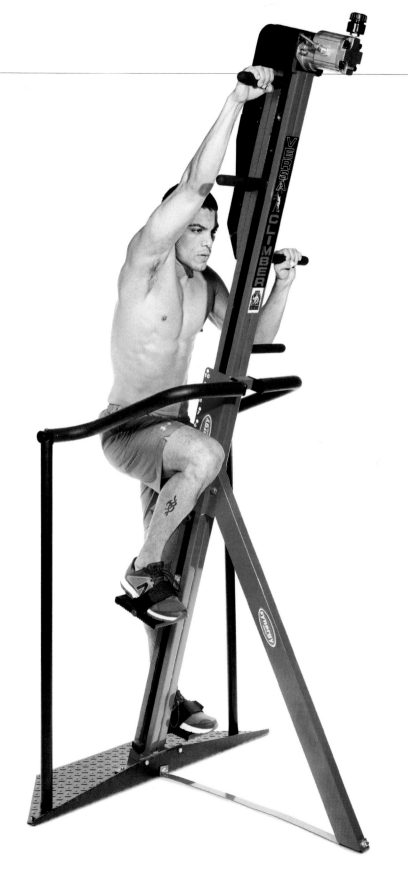

27 BODY-WEIGHT CARDIO

People often don't give weight training enough credit for its positive effect on the heart. It will raise your heart rate just as effectively as any cardio machine, while benefiting your muscles. Body-weight training works in much the same way, so if you're out of machines, just use the floor you're standing on.

THE BEST TOTAL-BODY CARDIO WORKOUT

WORKOUT #91   BY RAMONA BRAGANZA

A trainer to Hollywood celebrities, Ramona Braganza had to invent a system that would both get her clients ripped in short order and keep them engaged in their workouts. Her solution mixes cardio with body-weight circuits and core training for a three-pronged gut attack.

HOW IT WORKS Dubbed "321," as in three cardio intervals, two circuits, and one core exercise, it's not as easy as it sounds, even if the session does take only 20 minutes of your time. Follow the steps in order and keep your water handy.

DIRECTIONS There are three bouts of cardio (Cardio 1, 2, and 3), two circuits, and one core move. For the circuits, complete the exercises in succession and then rest 30 seconds before repeating once more.

CARDIO 1

Jog for two minutes.

▼ CIRCUIT 1

A OVERHEAD LUNGE

REPS: 10 (EACH SIDE)   REST: 0 SEC.

Raise your arms overhead and step forward with your right leg. Lower your body until your right thigh is parallel to the floor and your rear knee nearly touches the floor.

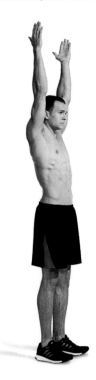
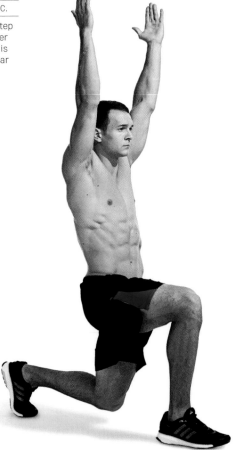

B SKYDIVER LUNGE

REPS: 12   REST: 0 SEC.

Get on the floor in the bottom of a pushup position. Push yourself up, then lower back down to rest your belly on the floor. Now raise your arms and legs up off the floor so you look like a skydiver in free fall. Place your hands and feet back down and push yourself back up. That's one rep.

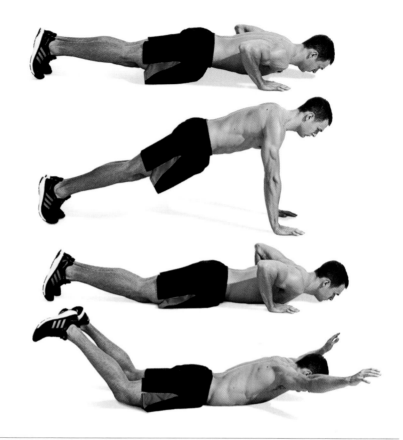

C GLUTE BRIDGE

REPS: 12   REST: 30 SEC.

Lie on your back on the floor with knees bent 90 degrees and heels on the floor. Extend your arms by your sides. Squeeze your glutes and push your heels into the floor to raise your hips until your torso and thighs form a line. Lower your hips until they're just above the floor.

REPEAT
CIRCUIT
ONCE
MORE

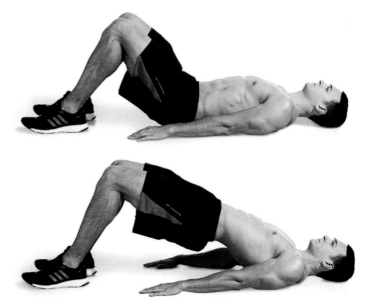

CARDIO 2

Shadowbox for two minutes. Throw punches with both hands, keep your guard up, and practice shuffling your feet forward, back, and side to side.

▼ CIRCUIT 2

A SUMO SQUAT

REPS: 15 REST: 0 SEC.

Stand with feet outside shoulder width and turn your toes out 45 degrees. Raise your arms up for balance. As you squat down, push your knees out and then drive your heels into the floor as you come up.

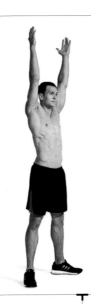
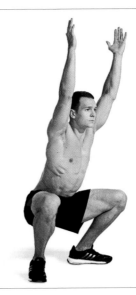

B PIKE PUSHUP

REPS: 12 REST: 0 SEC.

Get into pushup position with hands slightly wider than shoulder width. Push your body backward so your hips rise in the air and your torso points toward the floor. Keeping your legs straight, lower your body until the top of your head nearly touches the floor, and then press up.

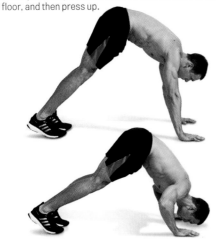

C FROG THRUST

REPS: 10 REST: 30 SEC.

Get into pushup position with feet wide apart. Hop your feet up to the outside of your hands so you look like you're about to leapfrog. Then hop them back again. That's one rep.

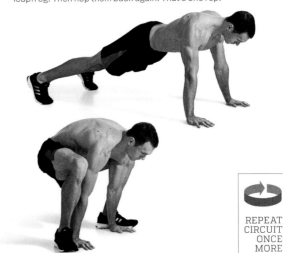

REPEAT CIRCUIT ONCE MORE

CARDIO 3

Go to a staircase and sprint or jog up it. Walk back down. Repeat for two minutes and mix it up—try skipping steps or hopping up the stairs.

▼ CORE

PLANK/SIDE PLANK COMBO

Get into pushup position and then lower your forearms to the floor. Hold 15 seconds, and then rotate your body to your right, resting on your left forearm and stacking your feet so your whole body faces 90 degrees to the floor. Hold 15 seconds. Rotate back to the floor and hold 15 seconds. Rotate to your left and hold the side plank again. Keep your hips elevated the whole time.

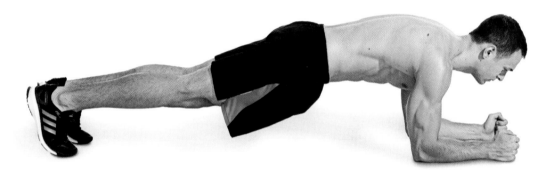

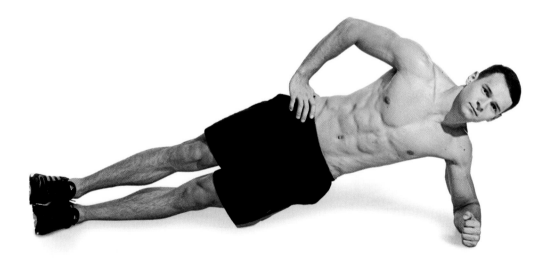

THE BEST SWIMMING WORKOUT

WORKOUT #92   BY GREGORY KINCHELOE

When trainers are asked to name the very "best" type of exercise, swimming regularly gets the top honor. There's no impact, it works every muscle in the body, and it makes your heart speed like an outboard motor. Whether you're looking to plunge into swimming because you want a body more like Ryan Lochte's, or you're already a swimmer in need of a new challenge in the pool, float this routine for a few weeks.

HOW IT WORKS The workout stresses good swim technique. Just practicing the basic strokes correctly will get the right muscles working in addition to helping you cut through the water faster and more efficiently (so you feel more like a fish in water than out). Over time, you'll reduce your rest periods to demand more of your heart and increase your potential for fat burning.

DIRECTIONS Perform the workout three times a week. Go by stroke cycles instead of distance—a sweep of each arm in turn is one cycle. If your pool is too small to complete the prescribed number of cycles in one direction, turn around quickly and continue to swim until the cycles are complete. After two weeks, reduce all rests by five seconds.

1 WARMUP

SETS: 4

Swim 12 stroke cycles at an easy pace. You can use the front crawl stroke or swim free-style. Rest a moment, then continue for three more sets.

2 50-YARD SWIM

SETS: 6 REST: 30 SEC.

Swim at a brisk pace for 50 yards, or 25 total stroke cycles.

3 FINGERTIP DRAG STROKE

SETS: 4 REST: 20 SEC.

Swim 12 stroke cycles, raising your elbows high out of the water as you reach for the next stroke so only your fingertips drag beneath the surface. Swim at a relaxed pace.

4 KICK DRILL

SETS: 4 REST: 30 SEC.

Grab a kickboard and rest your arms on it. Swim across the pool using only your legs. Do 25 kick cycles—one flutter of the left and right leg.

5 PULL DRILL

SETS: 6 REST: 20 SEC.

Hold the kickboard between your legs to keep them afloat, and swim using only your arms for 12 stroke cycles. Reach each arm far forward, but don't let your fingers come out of the water.

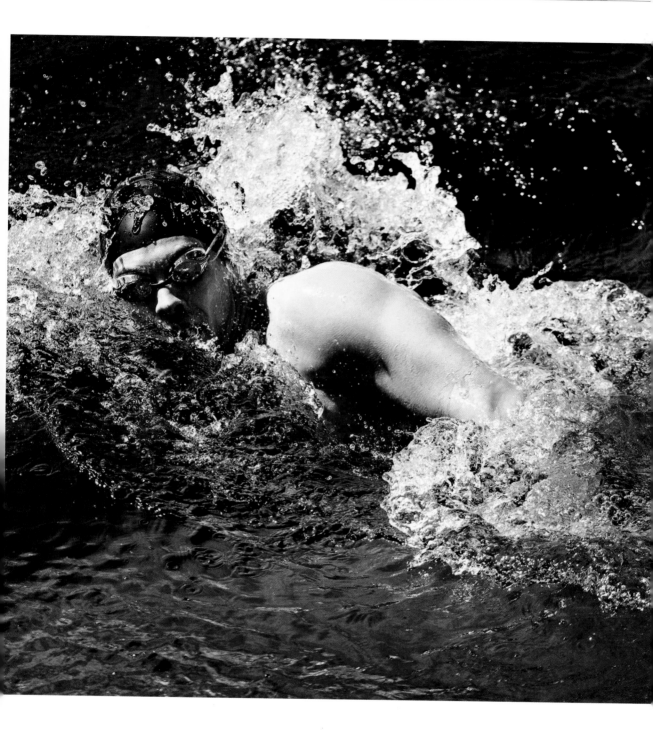

28

RUNNING

Running–either for food or for your life–is the oldest form of cardio, so we'd be remiss not to give it its own section. Whether you like to take it slow and steady or hit a top speed, either of these routines will lead you closer to a lean body with a healthier heart.

THE BEST
ENDURANCE-RUNNING WORKOUT

WORKOUT #93   BY STEVE GISSELMAN

As you may have gathered from all the interval and circuit workouts in this book, long, slow endurance training is not the best way to lose fat. So if you're thinking of starting a running program to get lean, we promise you'll do better with one of our strength-training options. Nevertheless, some people just enjoy running (maybe it's the endorphin rush known as "runner's high"?) and even aspire to compete in endurance races. If that's why you want to hit the trail, this program is especially for you.

HOW IT WORKS We've set up a seven-week routine to take you from a newbie runner (or someone who doesn't put in consistent road work) to an experienced one who's ready to take on a half marathon (13.1 miles). Most of the workouts are relatively short, so you can build your capacity gradually and avoid the knee pain and other overuse injuries associated with running too much, too soon. Brief workouts and plenty of built-in recovery time also allow you to live your life off the track—you don't have to rearrange everything around your training to make progress.

DIRECTIONS Follow the day-to-day running prescriptions for seven weeks.

WEEK 1

DAY 1
Run 1 mile at a 9:30 pace

DAY 2
Run 1 mile at a 9:00 pace

DAY 3
Off

DAY 4
Run 1 mile at a 9:30 pace
Rest 8 minutes
Repeat once more

DAY 5
Run 1 mile at a 9:30 pace
Rest 7 minutes
Run 1 mile at a 9:00 pace
Rest 7 minutes
Run 1 mile at a 9:30 pace

DAY 6
Off

DAY 7
Run 1 mile at a 9:00 pace

WEEK 2

DAY 8
Run 1 mile at an 8:30 pace

DAY 9
Off

DAY 10
Off

DAY 11
Run 1 mile at a 9:30 pace
Rest 6 minutes
Repeat twice more

DAY 12
Run 2 miles at a 9:30 pace
Rest 10 minutes

Repeat once more

DAY 13
Off

DAY 14
Run 400 meters at a 2:00 pace
Rest 2 minutes
Repeat three more times

WEEK 3

DAY 15
Run 200 meters at a 0:50 pace
Rest 2 minutes

DAY 16
Off

DAY 17
Run 1 mile at a 9:00 pace
Rest 5 minutes
Run 1 mile at an 8:30 pace
Rest 5 minutes
Run 1 mile at a 9:00 pace

DAY 18
Run 800 meters at a 4:15 pace
Rest 4 minutes
Repeat once more
Rest 7 minutes
Run 800 meters at a 4:05 pace
Rest 4 minutes
Repeat once more

DAY 19
Off

DAY 20
Off

DAY 21
Run 1 mile at an 8:30 pace
Rest 5 minutes
Run 1 mile at an 8:00 pace

WEEK 4

DAY 22
Run 800 meters at a 4:15 pace
Rest 60 seconds
Run 400 meters at a 1:50 pace
Rest 60 seconds
Run 200 meters at a 0:45 pace
Rest 60 seconds
Run 400 meters at a 1:45 pace
Rest 60 seconds
Run 200 meters at a 0:45 pace
Rest 60 seconds

DAY 23
Off

DAY 24
Run 1 mile at a 9:00 pace
Rest 5 minutes
Run 1 mile at an 8:30 pace
Rest 5 minutes
Run 1 mile at an 8:00 pace
Rest 5 minutes

DAY 25
Off

DAY 26
Run 100 meters at a 0:25 pace
Rest 90 seconds
Repeat four more times
Run 100 meters at a 0:22 pace
Rest 90 seconds
Repeat four more times

DAY 27
Off

DAY 28
Off

WEEK 5

DAY 29
Run 800 meters at a 4:05 pace
Rest 60 seconds
Run 400 meters at a 1:35 pace
Rest 60 seconds
Run 200 meters at a 0:40 pace
Rest 60 seconds
Run 400 meters at a 1:30 pace
Rest 60 seconds
Run 200 meters at a 0:40 pace
Rest 60 seconds

DAY 30
Off

DAY 31
Off

DAY 32
Run 1 mile at a 8:00 pace

DAY 33
Run 1 mile at a 7:45 pace

DAY 34
Off

DAY 35
Off

WEEK 6

DAY 36
Run 1 mile at an 8:30 pace
Rest 3 minutes
Run 1 mile at an 8:00 pace
Rest 4 minutes
Run 1 mile at an 8:00

DAY 37
Run 400 meters at a 0:90 pace
Rest 2 minutes
Repeat once more
Run 400 meters at a 0:95 pace
Rest 2 minutes
Repeat three more times

DAY 38
Off

DAY 39
Off

DAY 40
Run 2 miles at a 16:00 pace
Rest 8 minutes
Run 2 miles at a 16:00 pace

DAY 41
Run 200 meters at a 0:45 pace
Rest 90 seconds
Repeat seven more times

DAY 42
Run 1 mile at a 7:30 pace

WEEK 7

DAY 43
Off

DAY 44
Run 2 miles at a 15:00 pace

DAY 45
Off

DAY 46
Run 1 mile at a 7:30 pace

DAY 47
Off

DAY 48
Off

THE BEST SPRINT WORKOUT

WORKOUT #94   BY JASON FERRUGGIA

Sprinting may be the only kind of cardio that can be argued to build muscle as well as burn fat. Jason Ferruggia, designer of this workout and a longtime training adviser to *Men's Fitness*, is a huge fan of legendary NFL running back Walter Payton. He likes to point out that Payton, who was perpetually ripped and known for his durability, made hill sprints a cornerstone of his workouts throughout his career.

Do the same, and your pick-up game buddies may be calling you "Sweetness," or, at least, not "Slowness."

HOW IT WORKS Sprinting is intense exercise and can beat up your lower body if you don't ease into it. That's why we recommend doing it on a hill like Payton did, which will slow you down a bit so that you're less likely to pull a hamstring, quad, or hip flexor. Still, you'll work hard enough to raise testosterone and growth hormone levels—both associated with muscle growth—as well as improve speed and athleticism.

WARMUP

Warm up thoroughly beforehand and run a few practice sprints at a low intensity (but go a little faster each time).

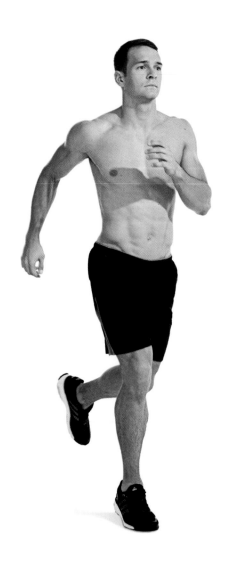

SPRINT

Perform 8 to 10 sprints of 20–40 yards. Run at slightly less than your absolute top speed for safety. Rest as needed between sets, but keep your heart rate elevated. Allow yourself enough recovery that you can go fast.

If you're new to sprinting or haven't done it in a while, do your sprints on a hill. Start with five and run only at a moderate pace and build up from there.

Land on the balls of your feet as you sprint, not your heels. Your front foot should land directly beneath you (unless the hill is especially steep). Your arms should pump vigorously forward and backward as you run. Let your hands come up to face level and then back to your pockets, but no further. Keep your shoulders and hips level so there's no side-to-side rotation in your torso.

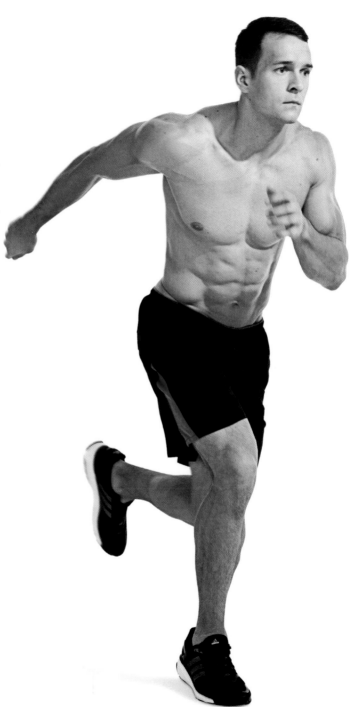

29

BOXING & MMA

Every guy wants to look like a fighter, before a fight, that is. The ripped, athletic look of a fighter says "strong," "capable," "explosive," but not "vain" or "musclebound." We talked to fighters and fight trainers to bring you the following boxing and MMA workouts, all designed to hit your gut hard.

THE BEST PUNCHING-BAG WORKOUT

WORKOUT #95   BY ZACH EVEN-ESH

Boxers, kickboxers, and mixed martial arts fighters don't use treadmills to get ripped. Their shredded physiques come from fight training, of which pounding a heavy bag is a major component. Dust off the one in your basement, lace up the gloves, and beat your gut once and for all.

HOW IT WORKS Hitting a bag builds punching power, stamina, and can increase your metabolic rate for days afterward. This workout involves your legs as well as your arms to train the whole body, activating as much muscle as possible to burn the most calories.

DIRECTIONS Perform the exercises as a circuit, completing one after the other without rest. Afterward, rest 30 seconds. That's one round. Repeat for five total rounds. To avoid injury, wear hand wraps and bag gloves.

1 LOW KICK - RIGHT LEG

REPS: 5 REST: 0 SEC.

Kick the lower half of the bag, as if aiming for an opponent's leg. Pivot on your support foot and turn your hip over as you deliver the kick, to maximize power. Complete five low kicks.

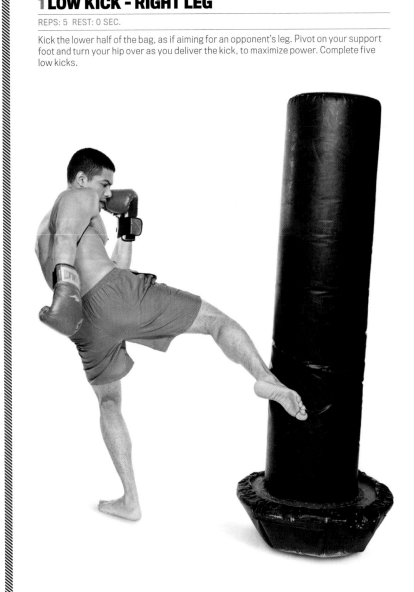

2 HIGH KICK - RIGHT LEG

REPS: 5 REST: 0 SEC.

Kick the upper half of the bag, as if aiming for an opponent's head. Keep your hands raised as if guarding your chin. Throw five kicks.

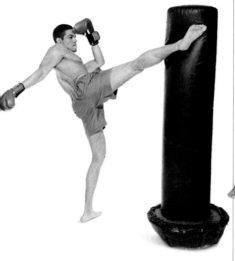

3 LOW KICK - LEFT LEG

REPS: 5 REST: 0 SEC.

Repeat the low kicks on the left leg.

4 HIGH KICK - LEFT LEG

REPS: 5 REST: 0 SEC.

Repeat the high kicks on the left leg.

5 PUNCHES

REPS: 20 REST: 0 SEC.

Perform 20 straight punches on the bag, alternating hands. Keep your guard up and turn your hips into each punch.

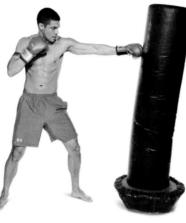

6 LEFT HOOK

REPS: 5 REST: 0 SEC.

Perform five left hooks—swing your arm in an arc to hit the side of the bag.

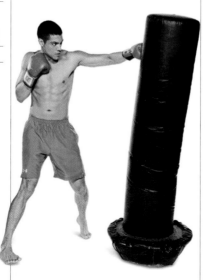

7 RIGHT HOOK

REPS: 5 REST: 0 SEC.

Perform five on the right side.

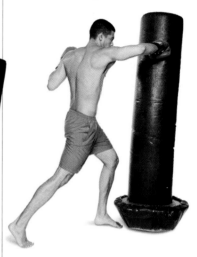

8 KNEE STRIKE

REPS: 5 REST: 30 SEC.

Drive one knee up into the bag. Repeat on the other leg.

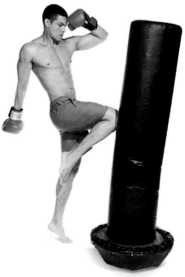

THE BEST
JUMP-ROPE WORKOUT

WORKOUT #96   BY MARTIN ROONEY, C.S.C.S.

Some time after grade school, guys stop jumping rope—unless they grow up to be boxers. But the jump rope may be the most portable and convenient cardio tool available. Relearn how to use it and you'll be lean, spry, and well conditioned for life.

HOW IT WORKS Make sure you've got a good rope. Beaded or plastic "speed" ropes are more durable than cotton ones and whip around faster, making for a more intense workout. They're also mandatory if you want to build up to doing advanced jump-rope moves like the double jump (which we've included here, although we don't expect you to master it right away). Before you begin using a rope, measure it to your height. When you stand on the middle of the rope, the handles should extend to your armpits. Cut and adjust the length as necessary.

You have to gradually prepare your lower body for the impact of jumping, so begin on a waxed wooden floor or rubber floor.

Hold the rope with hands at about hip height and elbows slightly bent, keeping your upper arms close to your sides. Your chest should be out and your shoulders back and down. Make your jumps small and land on the balls of your feet.

DIRECTIONS The workout consists of three training blocks. You'll practice different jumps, rest two minutes, and move on to the next block. Follow the instructions.

BLOCK 1

1 FORWARD JUMP

REPS: 60 SEC.

Jump over the rope with both feet on every revolution, swinging the rope forward (the most basic jump).

2 SIDE-TO-SIDE JUMP

REPS: 60 SEC.

Jump a few inches to your left as you swing the rope. Then to your right. Get into a rhythm.

3 BACKWARD JUMP

REPS: 60 SEC.

Swing the rope backward for each jump.

4 SINGLE-LEG JUMP - LEFT

REPS: 60 SEC.

Jump on one foot; land softly.

5 SINGLE-LEG JUMP - RIGHT

REPS: 60 SEC.

Jump on the other foot.

> REST
> 120 SEC.

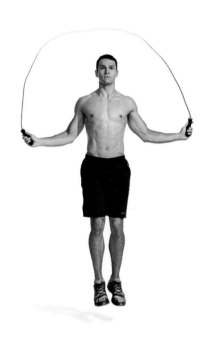
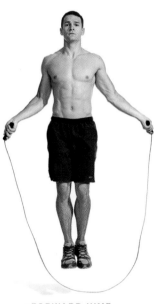

▲ FORWARD JUMP

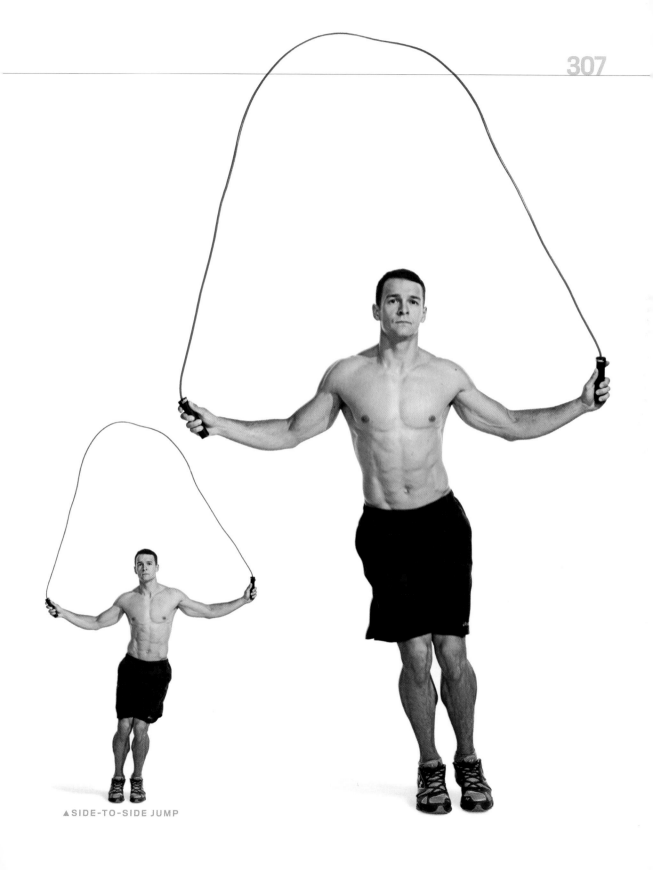

▲SIDE-TO-SIDE JUMP

BLOCK 2

1 FORWARD JUMP

REPS: 60 SEC.

2 ALTERNATING JUMP

REPS: 60 SEC.

Jump on one foot and then the other, back and forth.

3 FOOT-CROSS JUMP

REPS: 60 SEC.

Cross your feet over each other on each rep. Alternate the foot that lands in front.

4 SINGLE-LEG JUMP - LEFT

REPS: 60 SEC.

5 SINGLE-LEG JUMP - RIGHT

REPS: 60 SEC.

REST
120 SEC.

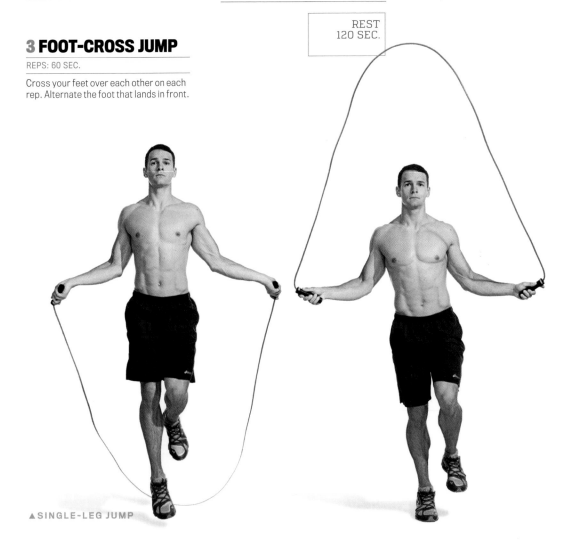

▲ SINGLE-LEG JUMP

BLOCK 3

1 FORWARD JUMP
REPS: 60 SEC.

3 BACKWARD JUMP
REPS: 60 SEC.

2 DOUBLE JUMP
REPS: 30 SEC.

Jump high enough that you can pass
the rope under your feet twice on every
revolution. If you can't do it fluidly, practice
it for 30 seconds—it doesn't matter how
many times you miss.

4 DOUBLE JUMP
REPS: 30 SEC.

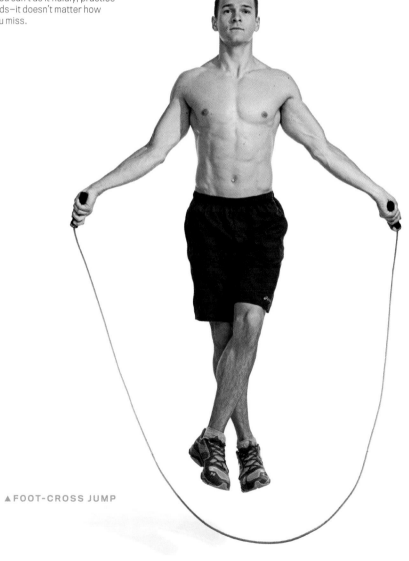

▲ FOOT-CROSS JUMP

THE BEST
MMA CARDIO WORKOUT

WORKOUT #97   BY MICHAEL SCHLETTER, C.P.T.

It's probably best that you leave mixed martial arts fighting to the professionals in the UFC and watch it from the safety of your couch (behind the bag of Fritos). But there's no reason you can't train like a fighter to lose fat and build your wind. The following is a pretty good simulation of an MMA fight—you know, without the foot about to land upside your head.

HOW IT WORKS The workout lasts approximately as long as a real championship MMA fight: five rounds. In those rounds you'll perform a little of nearly every kind of exercise that fighters use to prepare for battle, from jumping rope to bodyweight circuits to combinations on the heavy bag. Use it to get in fighting shape, and then watch the real fights from the safety of your couch.

DIRECTIONS Follow the instructions for the five rounds.

▼ ROUND 1

WARMUP, 3 MINUTES TOTAL WORK

Jump rope for three minutes; rest 90 seconds.

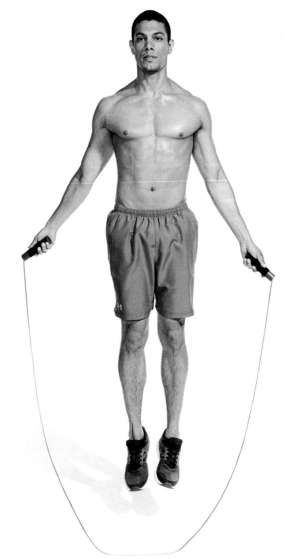

▼ **ROUND** 2

4 MINUTES TOTAL WORK

Shadowbox for two minutes. Then perform the circuit of exercises for two more minutes:

SHADOWBOX

Stay light on your feet and throw jabs, crosses, hooks, and uppercuts at an imaginary opponent. Keep your hands up.

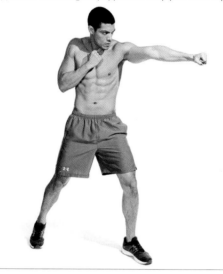

PUSHUP

Perform conventional pushups, aiming for 20 reps.

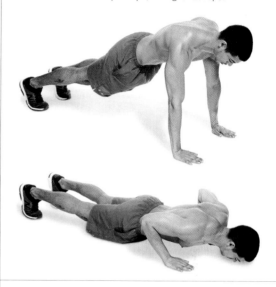

BODY-WEIGHT SQUAT

Stand with feet shoulder width and toes turned slightly out. Bend your hips back and squat as low as you can. Aim for 20 reps.

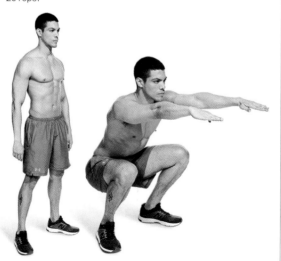

PLANK

Get into pushup position and then bend your elbows so your forearms lie flat on the floor. Brace your abs and hold the position until the end of two minutes.

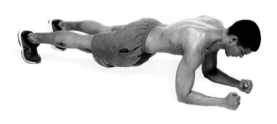

REST
90 SEC.

▼ ROUND 3

5 MINUTES TOTAL WORK

Perform the following combinations on the heavy bag and then jump rope for the remainder of five minutes.

50 JABS

50 CROSSES

50 JABS AND CROSSES

25 JABS, CROSSES, AND HOOKS

JUMP ROPE

> REST
> 120 SEC.

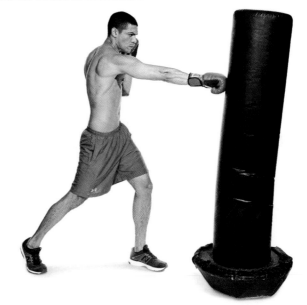

▼ ROUND 4

5 MINUTES TOTAL WORK

Perform the following combinations on a heavy bag and then jump rope for the remainder of five minutes.

ALTERNATING KNEE STRIKES, 60 SECONDS

ALTERNATING KICKS, 60 SECONDS

50 JABS AND KICKS

50 CROSSES AND KICKS

JUMP ROPE

> REST
> 120 SEC.

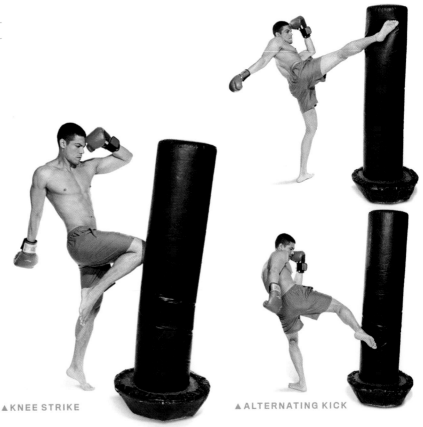

▲KNEE STRIKE   ▲ALTERNATING KICK

▼ ROUND 5

5 MINUTES TOTAL WORK

Perform the following grappling drills on the floor for five minutes.

10 FORWARD ROLLS
10 BACKWARD ROLLS
100 SITUPS
GROUND N' POUND
(place a heavy bag or shield on the floor; mount, and strike it)

15 PUSHUPS
JUMP ROPE

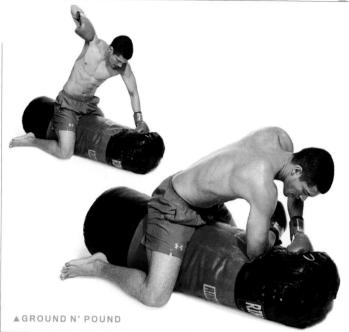

▲ GROUND N' POUND

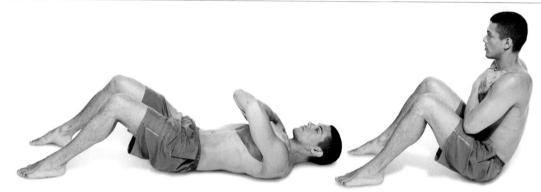

▲ SITUP

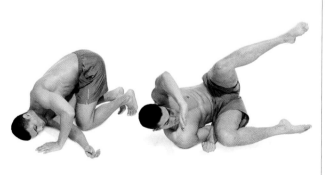

▲ FORWARD ROLL

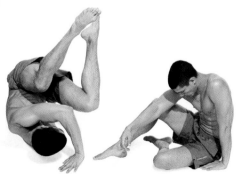

▲ BACKWARD ROLL

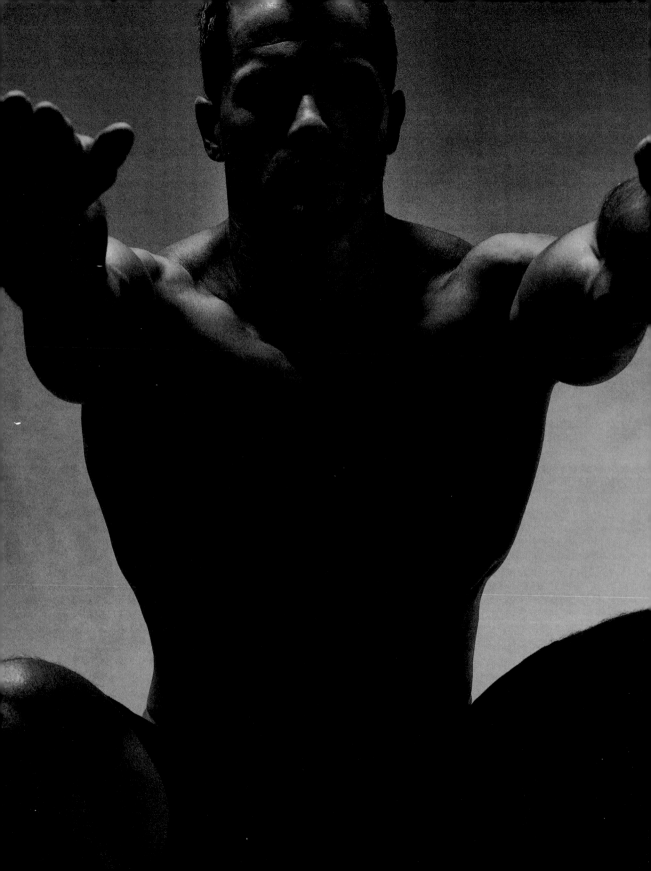

SHORT WORKOUTS

30 ABS IN UNDER 30 MINUTES

It doesn't take long to build muscles and burn fat. If the stimulus is intense, the time it takes to apply it can and should be very short. Depending on how dire your time constraints are, you can choose one of these workouts to let you sneak in some training. We offer routines for 30, 20, 10, and even just four minutes.

THE BEST 30-MINUTE WORKOUT

WORKOUT #98   BY JIM SMITH, C.S.C.S.

The best way to get more out of your workouts is to set a time limit for yourself. Racing the clock forces you to work harder, faster, and more efficiently. Every second counts. This is what Escalating Density Training (EDT)—as made famous by strength coach Charles Staley—is all about: Pick a duration and get the best workout possible before the clock runs out. You're about to find out how to use EDT to sculpt a great body when you have time for nothing less.

HOW IT WORKS Here's how EDT works. First, set a time limit—in this case, 30 minutes. Pick two different body parts you want to train that don't compete with each other; for example, chest and back or hamstrings and thighs. A pair like chest and shoulders would not work because it involves the same muscles and will fatigue you too fast.

Choose an exercise for each body part and a weight that allows you 10-12 reps for each. Begin alternating sets of the two moves, resting as little as possible between sets. Go a few reps short of failure on every set.

Continue until 30 minutes is up. Make note of the rest periods you took between sets and the total number of reps you performed. The next time you repeat the workout, try to improve your performance without extending the time frame. At right are examples of EDT supersets you can use.

▼ SUPERSET OPTIONS

SHOULDERS AND BACK
Dumbbell Overhead Press
Lat Pulldown

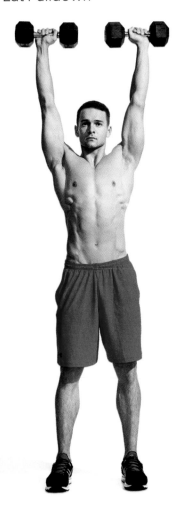

HAMSTRINGS AND THIGHS
Barbell Romanian Deadlift
Leg Extension

THIGHS AND CHEST
Front Squat
Pushup

BICEPS AND TRICEPS
Barbell Curl
Close-Grip Pushup

THIGHS AND BACK
Leg Press
Pullup

CHEST AND BACK
Dumbbell Bench Press
Seated Cable Row

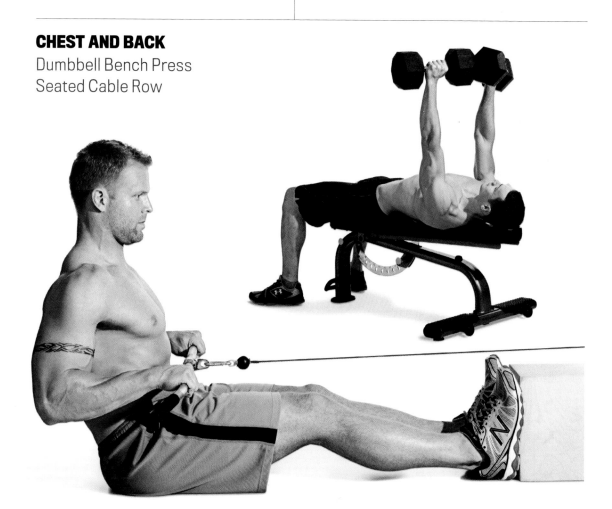

THE BEST
20-MINUTE WORKOUT

WORKOUT #99   BY MICHAEL CAMP, D.P.T., C.S.C.S.

Well-rounded fitness means being both strong and conditioned, but a tight schedule usually causes either weights or cardio to get left out of your program. The answer is to combine them both in one densely packed circuit.

HOW IT WORKS Although you'll train for only a fraction of the time that most guys sweat it out in gyms, you won't sacrifice big gains in this workout. The brisk pace will double as cardio, and the sequencing has another advantage as well—moving from smaller to larger muscle groups enhances the way your muscles are recruited, resulting in greater strength and muscle gains.

DIRECTIONS The workout is broken into six circuits. It may look long, but the whole routine will take only 20 minutes. Perform the circuits in order, repeating where noted. Your rest between exercises should be only as long as it takes to transition between moves. Repeat this workout up to four times a week on nonconsecutive days.

▼ CIRCUIT A

1 TREADMILL RUN/WALK

Walk one minute and then sprint one minute.

2 DUMBBELL FLYE

REPS: 8-10

Lie on a flat bench with a dumbbell in each hand. Keep a slight bend in your elbows as you spread your arms wide, lowering the weights until they're even with your chest. Flex your pecs and lift the weights back to the starting position.

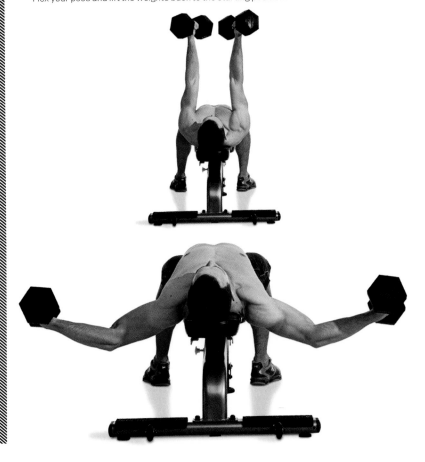

3 PUSHUP

REPS: NO MORE THAN 15

Place your hands on the floor at shoulder width. Keeping your abs braced and your body in a straight line, squeeze your shoulder blades together and lower your body until your chest is an inch above the floor.

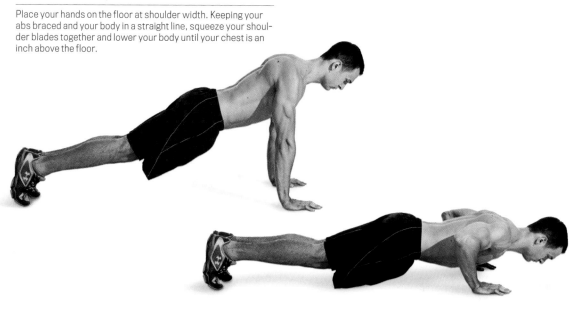

4 PLANK

REPS: 30 SEC.

Get into pushup position and then lower your forearms to the floor. Brace your abs and hold the position.

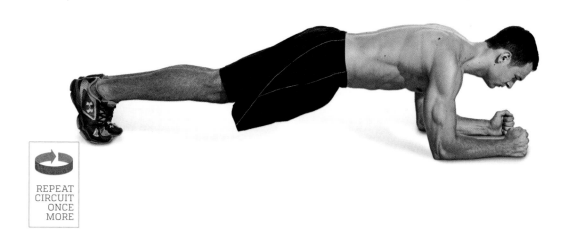

REPEAT
CIRCUIT
ONCE
MORE

▼ CIRCUIT B

1 PULLUP

REPS: AS MANY AS POSSIBLE

Hang from a pullup bar with hands facing
away from you outside shoulder width. Pull
yourself up until your chin is over the bar.

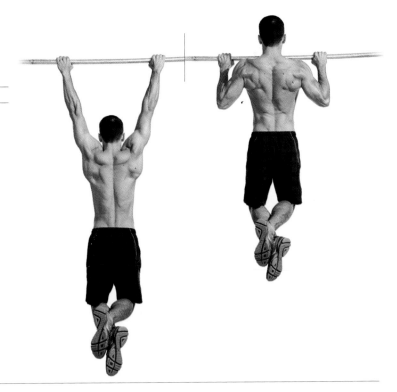

2 DUMBBELL LATERAL RAISE

REPS: 12-15

Hold a dumbbell in each hand and stand with
palms facing your sides. Raise the weights
up and out 90 degrees until your arms are
parallel to the floor.

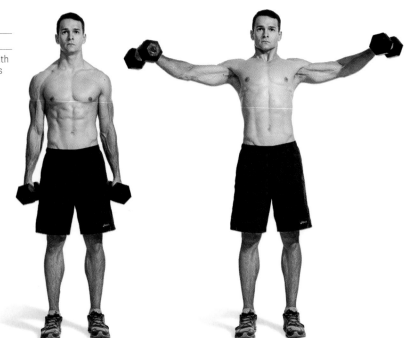

3 LYING DUMBBELL SKULL CRUSHER

REPS: 10-12

Lie back on a flat bench with a dumbbell in each hand. Hold the weights over your chest, palms facing each other. Bend your elbows and lower the weights to the sides of your head.

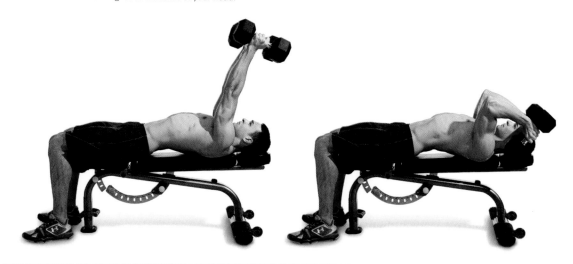

4 SIDE-TO-SIDE HOP

REPS: 30 SEC.

Place something small on the floor to act as a hurdle and jump over it side to side. Minimize your contact with the floor.

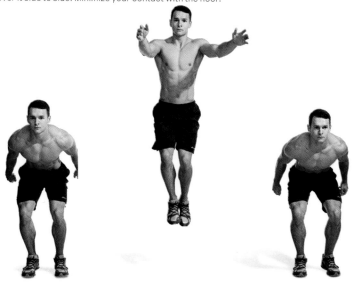

REPEAT
CIRCUIT
ONCE
MORE

▼ CIRCUIT C

1 DUMBBELL LUNGE

REPS: 20 (EACH LEG)

Stand with your feet hip width, holding a dumbbell in each hand. Step forward with one leg and lower your body until your rear knee nearly touches the floor and your front thigh is parallel to the floor.

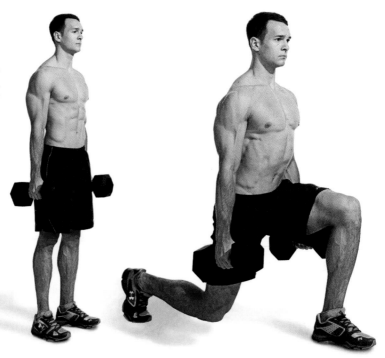

2 BURPEE

REPS: 10

Stand with feet shoulder width and bend down and place your hands on the floor. Now shoot your legs behind you fast so you end up in the top of a pushup position. Jump your legs back up so they land between your hands and then stand up quickly.

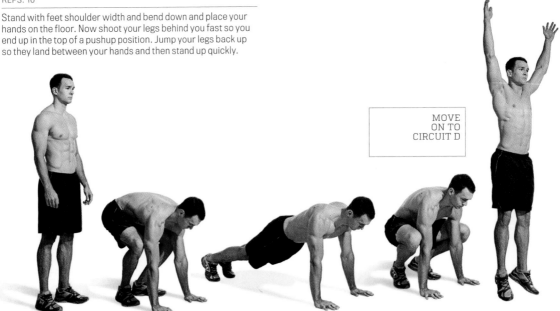

MOVE
ON TO
CIRCUIT D

▼ CIRCUIT D

1 DUMBBELL PULLOVER

REPS: 10

Lie on a bench holding a dumbbell by one end over your face. Lower the weight behind your head so you feel a stretch in your lats. Pull the weight back over your face.

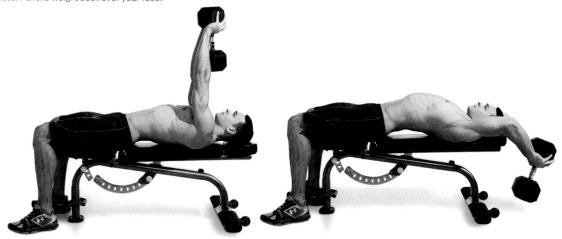

2 HOP ONTO BENCH

REPS: 20

Stand behind a bench or low box and hop up onto it. Step down and repeat.

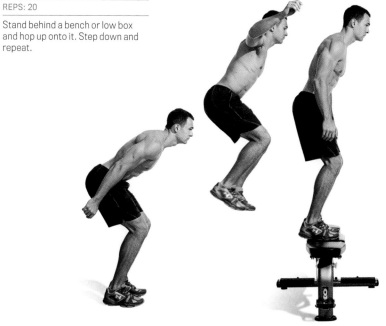

REPEAT
CIRCUIT
ONCE
MORE

▼ CIRCUIT E

1 DUMBBELL CURL

REPS: 15

Hold a dumbbell in each hand and, keeping your upper arms in place, curl the weights.

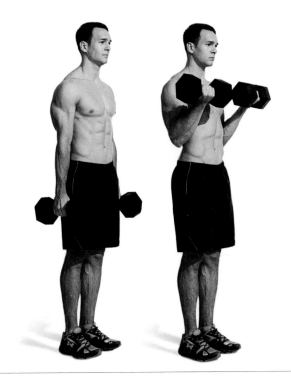

2 LATERAL BAND WALK

REPS: 20

Wrap an elastic band around your ankles and step sideways for 20 feet and then come back, keeping tension on your legs throughout.

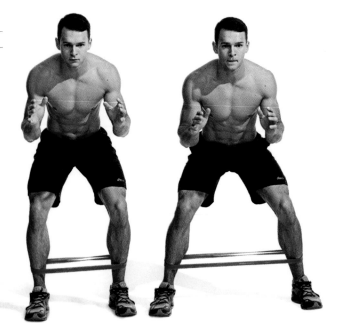

REPEAT CIRCUIT ONCE MORE

▼ CIRCUIT F

1 STEPUP

REPS: 30 SEC.

Place one foot on a bench or box, as shown. Step up onto the surface, but don't rest the trailing leg on it. Alternate legs each rep.

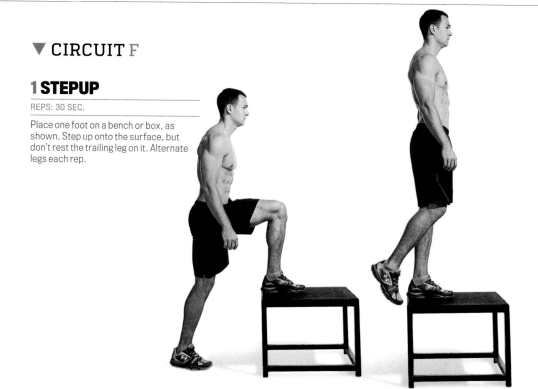

2 LEG LIFT

REPS: TO FAILURE

Lie on the floor and hold onto a bench or the legs of a heavy chair for support. Keep your legs straight and raise them up until they're vertical. Lower back down, but stop just short of the floor to keep tension on your abs before the next rep.

THE BEST ANYTIME WORKOUT

WORKOUT #100   BY JOE STANKOWSKI, C.P.T.

If you're the type of guy who makes excuses and misses workouts, you're going to hate this plan. But stick with it and you'll torch fat and improve your cardio in 10 minutes—wherever life has landed you at the moment.

HOW IT WORKS This routine works around your schedule and surroundings. Whether you have a lot of time or a little, you'll do as many reps of basic body-weight exercises as you can—no equipment or big open space required. By tracking your total number of reps, you'll be able to set goals and measure progress. Your mission must simply be to do more work in the next workout (of equal length) than you did in the previous one. This will ensure that your body is getting more efficient and better conditioned.

DIRECTIONS Set a timer for however long you have—even if you've got only 10 minutes. Complete as many reps as you can of each exercise, and count them. Stop a set when your form breaks down, and rest as needed. Make note of your total number of reps for the workout. Each time you repeat the workout with the same time period, try to complete more total reps.
   For example, if you worked out 10 minutes on Monday and then 25 minutes on Wednesday but could manage only 10 minutes again on Friday, try to get more work done in Friday's session than in Monday's. Try to perform the workout four to six times per week.

1 PRISONER SQUAT

Place your hands behind your head, interlacing your fingers. Stand with your feet shoulder width and your toes turned slightly out. Squat as low as you can.

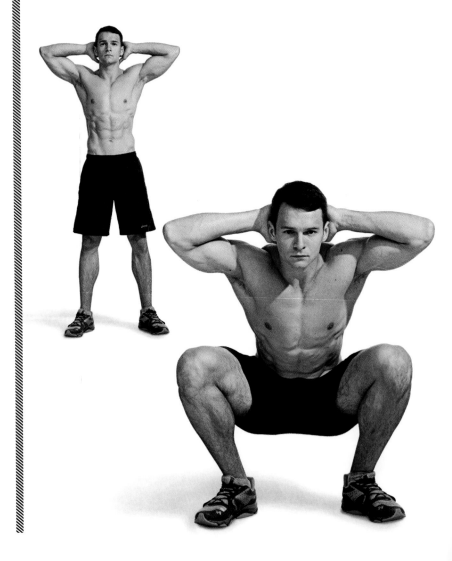

2 SEAL JUMP

Perform a jumping jack, reaching your arms out 90 degrees to your sides as your legs spread. When you jump your legs back in, clap your hands together in front of you.

3 PUSHUP

Place your hands on the floor at shoulder width. Keeping your abs braced and your body in a straight line, squeeze your shoulder blades together and lower your body until your chest is an inch above the floor.

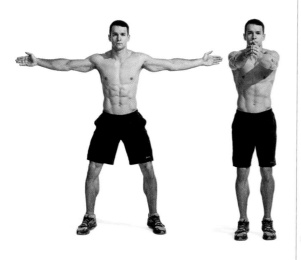

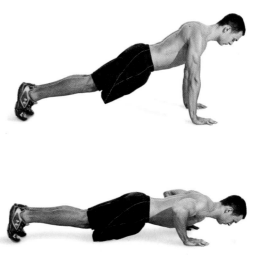

4 LATERAL JUMP

Jump to your right side and land on your right foot. Rebound off your right foot and jump back to your left to begin the next rep.

5 BURPEE

Stand with feet shoulder width and bend down and place your hands on the floor. Now shoot your legs behind you quickly so you end up in the top of a pushup position. Jump your legs back up so they land between your hands and then jump up in the air.

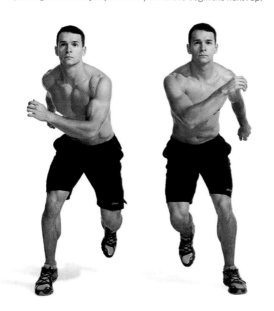

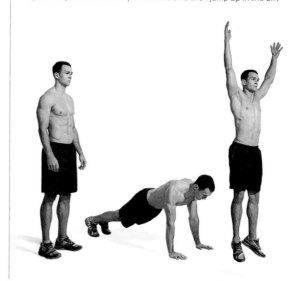

THE BEST
4-MINUTE WORKOUT

WORKOUT #101   BY SEAN HYSON, C.S.C.S.

Normally, we'd say that a workout that lasts four minutes must be wussy, but if it's a Tabata, that's another story. Izumi Tabata, Ph.D., a researcher at the National Institute of Fitness and Sports in Tokyo, Japan, found that brutally intense interval workouts lasting just four minutes improved endurance better than more conventional interval training—and increased fat burning. We know you've got the time for this workout, and to give you one less excuse to skip it, we'll give you only one exercise to do.

HOW IT WORKS Tabata workouts are designed according to a work-to-rest ratio of 2:1. You go as hard as you can for, say, 20 seconds, rest 10, and then repeat. You can choose one or several exercises to use for Tabatas. We've prescribed just the burpee. A total-body exercise equally favored and dreaded by martial artists and soldiers, the burpee tires you out faster than probably any other body-weight movement. It will make the ensuing four minutes the slowest of your life.

DIRECTIONS Perform burpees for 20 seconds. Don't worry about counting reps—just set a timer and do as many as you can. Then rest 10 seconds, and repeat for four minutes. Over time, you can add time to the work interval, but keep the ratio of work to rest at 2:1 (so if you build up to doing burpees for 30 seconds, rest 15 seconds between sets).

BURPEE

Stand with feet shoulder width and bend down and place your hands on the floor. Now shoot your legs behind you quickly so you're in the top of a pushup position. Jump your legs back up so they land between your hands and then jump up quickly.

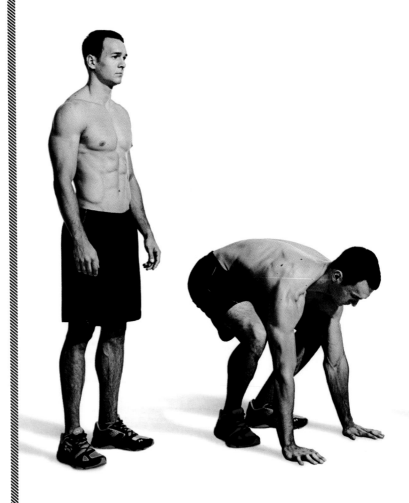

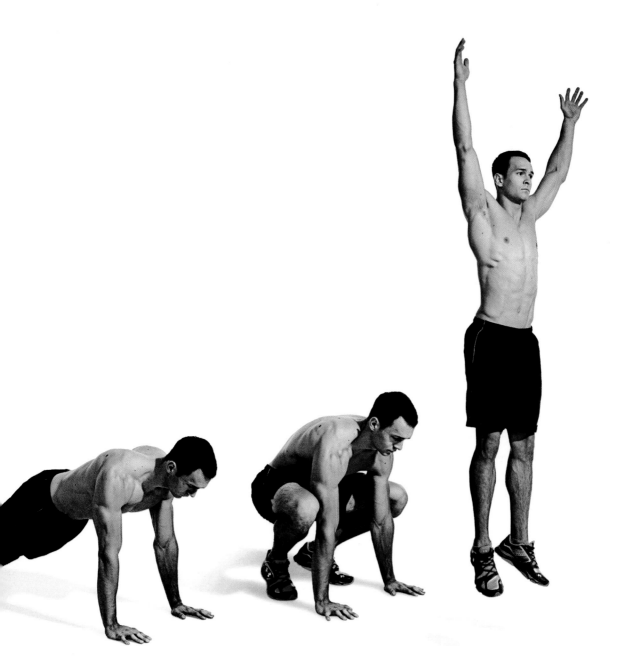

Page numbers in italics refer to illustrations.

A

abs, exercises for, 34-37, 40, 44-47, 50-51, 62-65, 80-81, 84-87, 89-91, 96, 152, 158, 162, 200, 237-51, 267, 290
> band-only, 242-43
> barbell-only, 240-41
> body-weight, 250-51
> full-gym, 238-39
> medicine-ball, 246-47
> Swiss-ball, 248-49
> in under 30 minutes, 315-29

Ab-Wheel Rollout, 239
All-Machine Workouts, 68-71
Alternating Dumbbell Bench Press, 42
Alternating Dumbbell Row, 41
Alternating Jump, 308
amino acids, 10
Ankle Mobilization, 219
> Wall, 240

anytime workouts, 326-27
Aquaman, 193
arms, exercises for, 34-37, 39-40, 103-11
> band-only, 107
> barbell-only, 106
> body-weight, 110-11
> dumbbell-only, 104-5
> suspension-trainer, 108-9
> see also biceps, exercises for; forearms, exercises for

Arms-High Partial Situp, 251

B

back, exercises for, 34-37, 91, 100, 101, 108, 126, 137, 138, 152, 154, 185-97, 267
> barbell-only, 188-89
> body-weight, 194-95
> dumbbell-only, 190-93
> full-gym, 186-87
> in short workouts, 316, 317
> suspension-trainer, 196-97
> see also chinup(s); rowing machines

Back Extension, 187
> Prone, 192
> Reverse, 233
> Single-Leg, 201
> Weighted, 271

Backward Jump, 306, 309
Backward Roll, 313
Backward Sprint, 97
Band Curl, 107
band-only workouts:
> for abs, 242-43
> for arms, 107
> for biceps, 120-21
> for chest, 160-61
> full-body, 73-77
> for shoulders, 172-75
> for triceps, 132-33

Band Pushdown, 107, 125
Band-Resisted Flye, 161
Band-Resisted Pushup with Feet Elevated, 161
Barbell Calf Raise, 206
Barbell Curl, 317
Barbell Glute Bridge, 228
Barbell Hip Thrust, 224
barbell-only workouts:
> for abs, 240-41
> for arms, 106
> for back, 188-89
> for biceps, 116-17
> for butt, 226-29
> for chest, 150-51
> for forearms, 142-43
> full-body, 49-53
> for legs, 204-7
> for shoulders, 170-71
> for traps, 254-55
> for triceps, 126-27

Barbell Rollout, 241
Barbell Romanian Deadlift, 317
Barbell Russian Twist, 51
Bear Crawl, 96
Behind-the-Back Cable Curl, 115
Bench Press, 36, 123, 147, 150, 262
> Alternating Dumbbell, 42
> Close-Grip, 124
> Dumbbell, 27, 147, 317
> Incline, 261

Incline Dumbbell, 39, 148
Incline Neutral Grip, 31
Low-Incline, 150
Neutral-Grip Dumbbell, 27, 128
Smith Machine Incline, 146
Speed, 151
Bentover Lateral Raise, 57, 174
Bentover Lateral Raise-Thumbs Up, 257
Bentover Reverse Flye, 191
Bentover Row, 45, 193
to Neck, 189
Bentover YTW, 15
biceps, exercises for, 34-37, 105, 106, 108-9, 110-11, 113-21, 138, 142, 196
band-only, 120-21
barbell-only, 116-17
dumbbell-only, 118-19
full-gym, 114-15
in short workouts, 317
see also chinups; rowing exercises
Biceps Curl, 77, 109
on suspension trainer, 197
Biceps/Triceps Stretch, 107
bikes, stationary, 273
workout for, 282-83
Bird Dog, 16
Blurpee, 100, 101
body-part workouts, 103-256
for abs, 237-51, 315-29
for arms, 103-11
for back, 185-97
for biceps, 113-21
for butt, 223-35
for calves, 215-21
for chest, 145-63
for forearms, 137-43
for legs, 199-213
for shoulders, 165-83
for traps, 253-57
for triceps, 123-35
body recomposition workouts, 26-33
Body-Weight Calf-Raise, 207
Body-Weight Squat, 91, 311

body-weight workouts:
for abs, 250-51
for arms, 110-11
for back, 194-95
for butt, 234-35
for calves, 220-21
cardio, 289-95
for chest, 162-63
4-minute, 328-29
full-body, 93-101
for legs, 208-11
for shoulders, 178-81
for triceps, 134-35
Boxing and MMA workouts, 303-12
Box Squat, 270
Braganza, Ramona, 290
Bruno, Ben, 208
Bulgarian Split Squat, 28, 58, 87, 213, 226, 231
Iso Hold, 211
1 1/2, 271
Burpee, 322, 327, 328
Burpee/Broad Jump, 98
butt, exercises for, 223-35
barbell-only, 226-29
body-weight, 234-35
full-gym, 224-25
suspension-trainer, 230-31
Swiss-ball, 232-33
Butterfly Hip Thrust, 233

C
Cable Crossover, 147
Cable Row:
Seated, 36, 187, 317
Towel, 138
Calf Raise on Leg Press, 71
Calf Stretch, 18
calories, 6, 8
burning of, 40, 44, 74, 84
calves, exercises for, 18, 34-37, 70, 206-7, 215-21
body-weight, 220-21
dumbbell-only, 218-19
full-gym, 216-17

see also Deadlift; squat(s)

carbohydrates, 6, 9, 10

cardio workouts, 273-313, 318
    body-weight, 289-95
    boxing and MMA, 303-12
    jump-rope, 306-9
    on machines, 273-87
    running, 297-301
    swimming, 294

cards, deck of, 134

Cat/Camel, 16

Cheat Curl, 119

chest, exercises for, 34-37, 90, 108, 145-63
    band-only, 160-61
    barbell-only, 150-51
    body-weight, 162-63
    dumbbell-only, 152-53
    full-gym, 146-49
    medicine-ball, 158-59
    in short workouts, 317
    suspension-trainer, 154-57

Chest Press, 68
    Hammer Strength, 149

Chest-Supported Row, 69

Chinup(s), 34, 47, 111, 186, 187, 195
    Close-Grip, 195
    Eccentric, 110, 111
    Fly-Away, 196
    Neutral Grip, 30

Circles, 244
    Elbow, 249

Clean and Press, 84, 170

Close-Grip Bench Press, 124

Close-Grip Chinup, 195

Close-Grip Curl, 117

Close-Grip Floor Press, 126

Close-Grip Pushup, 86, 100, 110, 133, 159, 317

Conventional Curl, 117

Cook Hip Lift, 234

core, exercises for, 50-51, 62-65, 80-81, 89-91, 96, 152, 158, 162, 200, 237-51, 290
    see also abs, exercises for

Crab Walk, 97

Crossover Pushup, 159

Crunch, 249
    Legs-On-Ball, 249
    Resisted Reverse, 243

Curl(s), 118, 123
    Band, 107
    Barbell, 317
    Behind-the-Back Cable, 115
    Bicep, 77, 109, 197
    Cheat, 119
    Close-Grip, 117
    Conventional, 117
    Drag, 119
    Dumbbell, 324
    EZ-Bar, 39
    EZ-Bar Reverse Preacher, 115
    Fat-Grip Hammer, 114
    Hammer, 105, 119
    Hammer Cheat, 140
    Hamstring, 232
    High-Speed, 120, 121
    Leg, 91, 213
    Poundstone, 106
    Reverse, 116, 121, 143
    Reverse Wrist, 141
    Seated, 104
    Seated Incline Dumbbell, 29
    Seated Zottman, 32
    Side, 121
    Towel, 142
    Towel Kettlebell, 139
    Wide-Grip, 117
    Wrist, 141
    Zottman, 32, 265

Cutler, Jay, 146

D

Deadlift, 26, 45, 137, 186
    Barbell Romanian, 317
    Dumbbell Romanian, 37, 41
    Rack, 255
    Romanian, 31, 52, 269
    Shrug Combo, 257

Single-Leg Romanian, 47, 56, 235
Snatch-Grip Rack, 42
Suitcase, 241
Sumo Romanian, 228
Trap-Bar, 38
Walking Single-Leg, 225
Decline EZ-Bar Lying Triceps Extension, 39
Decline EZ-Bar Triceps Extensions, 33
Decline Triceps Extension, 125
deltoid muscles, 170, 176, 190, 196
Diamond Pushup, 104
    with Cards, 134
diet, 5-11, 62
Dip, 29, 95, 132, 149, 180, 261
    Half, 135
Dip/Leg Raise, 99, 238
Double-Band Triceps Extension, 133
Double Jump, 309
Drag Curl, 119
Drop N' Pop, 159
dropsets, 194, 262
Dumbbell Bench Press, 147, 317
    Incline, 39, 148
    Neutral-Grip, 27
Dumbbell Curl, 324
    Seated Incline, 29
Dumbbell Flye, 149, 318
    Standing, 167
Dumbbell High Pull, 41
Dumbbell Lateral Raise, 264, 320
Dumbbell Lunge, 43, 322
dumbbell-only workouts:
    for arms, 104-5
    for back, 190-93
    for biceps, 118-19
    for calves, 218-19
    for chest, 152-53
    for forearms, 140-41
    full-body, 55-65
    for legs, 202-3
    for shoulders, 182-83
    for traps, 256-57
    for triceps, 128-31

Dumbbell Overhead Press, 59, 316
Dumbbell Pullover, 323
Dumbbell Pushup with Row, 57
Dumbbell Romanian Deadlift, 37, 41
Dumbbell Row, 263
    Alternating, 41
    Elbow-Out, 59
    Incline, 39
    One-Arm, Elbow-In, 60
Dumbbell Side Bend, 271
Dumbbell Squat, 59, 203
Dumbbell Stepup, 202

E
Eccentric Chinup, 110, 111
Elbow Circles, 249
Elbow-Out Dumbbell Row, 59
Elite, 73
elliptical machines, 273, 274
    workout for, 278
endurance-running workout, 298-99
Escalating Density Training (EDT), 316
European Journal of Applied Physiology, 10
EZ-Bar Curl, 39
EZ-Bar Reverse Preacher Curl, 115

F
Face Pull, 167
Farmer's Walk, 140, 256
"Fascia Stretch Training," 146
fascia tissue, 146
fat, 6, 9, 10
Fat-Grip Hammer Curl, 114
fat-loss workouts, 40-47, 62, 75
Feet-On-Ball Hip Thrust, 232
Ferriss, Tim, 100
Ferruggia, Jason, 20, 300
Figurehead, 231
Fingertip Drag Stroke, 294
Floor Press, 152
    Close-Grip, 126
    Lever, 51
    Neutral-Grip, 263
Flutter Kick, 251

Fly-Away Chinup, 196
flye exercises, 145, 152, 154
    Band-Resisted Flye, 161
    Bentover Reverse Flye, 191
    Dumbbell Flye, 149, 318
    Incline Dumbbell Flye, 147
    Prone Flye, 153
    Rear-Delt, 177
    Standing Dumbbell Flye, 167
    3-Way Flye, 154
Foot-Cross Jump, 308, 309
forearms, exercises for, 34-37, 96, 97, 128, 137-43
    barbell-only, 142-43
    dumbbell-only, 140-41
    full-gym, 138-39
Forward Jump, 306, 308, 309
Forward Sprint, 97
4-minute workout, 328-29
Frog Thrust, 292
Front Raise, 174
Front Squat, 30, 53, 240, 317
Front Squat to Press, 41
fruits, 9, 10
FST-7 method, 146
full-body workouts, 23-101
    band-only, 73-77
    barbell-only, 49-53
    for body recomposition, 26-33
    body weight, 93-101
    dumbbell/kettlebell, 55-65
    for fat loss, 40-47
    machine, 67-71
    medicine ball, 83-87
    for muscle, 34-39
    suspension trainer, 79-81
    Swiss ball, 89-91
full-gym workouts, 25-47
    for abs, 238-39
    for back, 186-87
    for biceps, 114-15
    for butt, 224-25
    for calves, 216-17
    for chest, 146-49
    for forearms, 138-39
    for legs, 200-201
    for shoulders, 166-69
    for triceps, 124-25

G
German Body Comp, 26, 30
Getup, Turkish, 64
glucose, 9
Glute Bridge, 231, 291
    Barbell, 228
    Single-Leg, 211, 212, 230, 233
    Walkout, 210
glutes, exercises for, 34-37, 202, 210, 211, 212, 223, 224, 226, 228, 230, 232, 233, 291
    see also butt, exercises for; legs, exercises for
Good Morning, 75
Grip Crush, 141
Groiner, 16
Ground N' Pound, 313
gyms, xiv, xv, 25, 67
    see also full-gym workouts
gym towels, as handle, 138, 142

H
Half Dip, 135
Half-Kneeling Cable Chop, 33
Half-Kneeling Chop, 243
Half-Kneeling Lift, 243
Hammer Cheat Curl, 140
Hammer Curl, 105, 119
    Fat-Grip, 114
Hammer Strength Chest Press, 149
Hammer Strength equipment, 67
Hamstring Curl, 232
hamstrings, exercises for, 34-37, 200, 202, 232
    in short workouts, 317
    see also Deadlift; legs, exercises for; squat(s)
Hang Clean, 45, 53, 188
Hard-Style Kettlebell Swing, 63
Heath, Phil, 146
High Kick-Left Leg, 305
High Kick-Right Leg, 305
High Pull, 168

Dumbbell, 41
  Snatch-Grip, 171, 254
High-Speed Curl, 120, 121
Hindu Pushup, 178
Hip Circles, 16
Hip Flexor Stretch, 17
Hip Hinge, 15
Hole Calf Raise, 221
Hop Onto Bench, 323
Horizontal Cable Woodchop, 44
Hyson, Sean, xv

I

Incline Bench Press, 261
Incline Dumbbell Flye, 147
Incline Dumbbell Press, 39, 148
Incline Dumbbell Row, 39
Incline Neutral-Grip Bench Press, 31
injuries, 67, 165, 200
  preventing of, 13, 23, 154, 160, 199, 298, 300
insulin, 9
Inverted Row, 28, 43
  Rotational, 109
  on suspension trainer, 156, 197

J

Jumping Calf Raise, 221
Jumping Jack, 218
jump-rope workout, 36-39
Jump Squat, 94, 205, 208
Jungle Gym XT, 79, 80

K

Kettlebell, towel curl with, 139
Kettlebell Press-Out, 63
kettlebell workouts, 55-65
Kick Drill, 294
Kneeling Hip Flexor Mobilization, 209, 227
Knee Strike, 305, 312

L

Landmine One-Arm Row, 189
Landmine Press, 151
Lateral Band Walk, 324

Lateral Jump, 327
Lateral Plank Walk, 181
Lateral Raise, 173
  Bentover, 57, 174, 257
  Dumbbell, 264, 320
  Lying, 187
Lat Pulldown, 316
lats, 100, 101, 106, 188, 190, 196
  see also back, exercises for
Lat Stretch, 17, 180
Left Hook, 305
Leg Curl, 91, 213
Leg Lift, 325
Leg Press, 71, 317
  Calf Raise on, 71
Leg Raise, 250
  Dip, 99, 238
legs, exercises for, 91, 96, 97, 199-213
  barbell-only, 204-7
  body-weight, 208-11
  dumbbell-only, 202-3
  full-gym, 200-201
  in short workouts, 317
  suspension-trainer, 212-13
  see also calves, exercises for
Legs-On-Ball Crunch, 249
Lever Floor Press, 51
Lock-Off, 158
Low-Cable Crossover, 149
lower-body workouts, 267-71
Low-Incline Press, 150
Low Kick-Left Leg, 305
Low-Kick-Right Leg, 304
Lunge, 100
  Dumbbell, 43, 322
  One-Arm Deficit Reverse, 225
  Overhead, 53, 290
  with Overhead Press, 57
  Reverse, 203
  Single-Arm Row with Partial, 51
  Single-Leg Wobble, 80
  Skydiver, 291
  Walking, 201, 211, 269

Lying Dumbbell Skull Crusher, 321
Lying Lateral Raise, 187
Lying Triceps Extension, 127, 129

M

machine workouts:
    cardio, 273-87
    elliptical, 278
    full-body, 67-71
    rowing machine, 280
    spin bike, 282-83
    stairclimber, 284
    treadmill, 276
    versaclimber, 286
macronutrients, 6
maximum heart rate (MHR), estimating of, 278
Meadows, John, 6, 9, 10
Meathead's Warmup, 19-20
Medicine-Ball Russian Twist, 239
medicine-ball workouts:
    for abs, 246-47
    for chest, 158-59
    full-body, 83-87
Men's Fitness Food Pyramid, 3, 6-11, 6
Miyaki, John, 6, 10
MMA cardio workout, 310-13
Mohr, Chris, 6
Mountain Climber, 86
muscles:
    chain of, 196
    deltoid, 170, 190, 196
    diet for building of, 6, 8
    flexing of, 146, 179
    stretching of, 14-18, 105, 160, 179, 180
    triset, 178
    see also specific muscles

N

neck muscles, exercises for, 253-57
    see also traps, exercises for
Neutral-Grip Chinup, 30
Neutral-Grip Dumbbell Bench Press, 27, 128
Neutral-Grip Floor Press, 263
Neutral-Grip Overhead Press, 182

Neutral-Grip Press, 128
Neutral-Grip Pulldown, 70
Neutral-Grip Triceps Extension, 105
nutrition, 6
    for workouts, 10

O

obesity, 6
1 1/2 Bulgarian Split Squat, 271
1 1/4 Neutral-Grip Dumbbell Bench Press, 27
1.5 Walking Lunge, 211
One-Arm, Elbow-In Dumbbell Overhead Press, 60
One-Arm, Elbow-In Dumbell Row, 60
One-Arm Deficit Reverse Lunge, 225
One-Arm Neutral-Grip Row, 190
One-Arm Overhead Extension, 131
One-Arm Snatch, 62
One-Arm Underhand Row, 192
One-Dumbbell/Kettlebell Workout, 62-65
Overhead Extension, One-Arm, 131
Overhead Lunge, 53, 290
Overhead Press, 35, 46, 53, 166, 241, 260
    with band, 172
    Dumbbell, 59, 316
    Lunge with, 57
    Neutral-Grip, 182
    One-Arm, Elbow-In Dumbbell, 60
Overhead Squat, 15

P

Pallof Press, 76, 242
Pallof Press Iso Hold, 37
Parallel Bar Hand Walk, 97
Pause Squat, 200
Payton, Walter, 300
pecs, 18, 145, 148, 150, 152, 154, 158, 162
    see also chest, exercises for
Pec Stretch, 18
Pike Press, 180
Pike Pushup, 176, 292
Pike-Up, 245
    to Superman, 91
Piriformis Stretch, 18
Plank(s), 163, 311, 319

Lateral Plank Walk, 181
  Side, 56, 247
  /Side Plank Combo, 293
  Star, 251
  Swiss Ball, 40
plateaus, 154
Plate Pressout, 153
Plyo Pushup, 160
Poundstone, Derek, 106
Poundstone Curl, 106
practical warmup, 21-22
Prisoner Squat, 326
Prone Back Extension, 192
Prone Flye, 153
protein, 6-9, 10
Pull Apart, 75
Pull Drill, 294
Pullover, 126, 127, 153
  Dumbbell, 323
  Triceps Extension, 106
Pullup(s), 94, 95, 138, 185, 261, 317, 320
  Knee Raise, 99
  Towel, 139
  Weighted, 35
  Wide-Grip, 194
Puncher's Pushup, 247
Punches, 305
punching-bag workout, 304-5
Push Press, 45
Pushup(s), 61, 162, 311, 317, 319, 327
  with band, 74, 161
  Band-Resisted, with Feet Elevated, 161
  Close-Grip, 86, 100, 110, 133, 159, 317
  Crossover, 159
  Diamond, 104
  Dumbbell Pushup with Row, 57
  with Feet on Ball, 90
  Hindu, 178
  with medicine ball, 84, 86, 158-59
  Pike, 176, 292
  Plyo, 160
  Puncher's, 247
  Rocket, 81
  on suspension trainer, 108, 156
  Wide-Grip, 161

Q

quads, exercises for, 34-37, 200, 202
  see also Deadlift; legs, exercises for; squat(s)

R

Rack Deadlift, 255
  Snatch-Grip, 42
Raise Complex, 183
Rambie, Hala, 26
Rambod, Hany, 146
Rear-Delt Flye, 177
reps, workout, 56, 68, 94, 98, 104, 116, 118, 120, 132, 150, 158, 162, 166, 186, 196, 216, 246, 250, 260, 262, 268
  deck of cards for, 134
Resisted Reverse Crunch, 243
Reverse Back Extension, 233
Reverse Curl, 116, 121, 143
  21, 143
Reverse Lunge, 203
  One-Arm Deficit, 225
Reverse Table-Up, 235
Reverse Wrist Curl, 141
Right Hook, 305
Rollout, 248
  Ab-Wheel, 239
  Barbell, 241
  Swiss-ball, 29
Romanian Deadlift, 31, 52, 269
  Barbell, 317
  Dumbbell, 37, 41
  Single-Leg, 47, 56, 235
  Sumo, 228
  Walking Single-Leg, 225
Rotational Inverted Row, 109
Roussell, Mike, 6
rowing machines, 273, 274
  workout for, 280
running workouts, 297-301
Russian Twist, 247
  Medicine-Ball, 239

S

saturated fat, 10

Seal Jump, 219, 327

Seated Band Row, 76

Seated Cable Row, 36, 187, 317

Seated Calf Raise, 217

    -Toes In, 219

    -Toes Neutral, 219

    -Toes Out, 218

Seated Curl, 104

Seated Dumbbell Clean, 169, 183, 264

Seated Incline Dumbell Curl, 29

Seated Knee Tuck, 87

Seated Zottman Curl, 32

Shadowbox, 311

short workouts, 315-29

    for anytime, 326-27

    4-minute, 328-29

    20-minute, 318-25

    30-minute, 316-17

Shoulder Over and Back, 14

Shoulder Press, 70

shoulders, exercises for, 34-35, 90-91, 108, 152, 154, 165-83, 197

    band-only, 172-75

    barbell-only, 170-71

    body-weight, 178-81

    dumbbell-only, 182-83

    full-gym, 166-69

    in short workouts, 316

    suspension-trainer, 176-77

Shoulder Stretch, 178

Shrug, 175

Side Curl, 121

Side Lunge, 15

Side-Lying Clam, 229

Side Plank, 247

    with Lateral Raise, 56

    Plank Combo, 293

Side-to-Side Hop, 321

Side-to-Side Jump, 306, 307

Single-Arm Row with Partial Lunge, 51

Single-Leg Back Extension, 201

Single-Leg Calf Raise, 220

Single-Leg Glute Bridge, 211, 212, 230, 233

Single-Leg Jumps, 306, 308

Single-Leg Romanian Deadlift, 47, 56, 235

Single-Leg Row, 80

Single-Leg Wobble Lunge, 80

Situp, 313

    Arms-High Partial, 251

    with Medicine-Ball Throw, 239

    Sprinter, 271

    Straight-Leg Barbell, 241

    and Throw, 85

    Weighted, 269

Skater Squat, 210

Skydiver Lunge, 291

Slam, 246

Smith Machine Incline Press, 146

Snatch-Grip High Pull, 171, 254

Snatch-Grip Low Pull, 255

Snatch-Grip Rack Deadlift, 42

Snatch-Grip Shrug Pull, 255

speed, building of, 84

Speed Bench Press, 151

"speed" ropes, 306

speed work, 150

spin bikes, 273, 274

    workout of, 282-83

Split Squat to Press, 50

Sprint:

    Backward, 97

    Forward, 97

Sprinter, 245

Sprinter Situp, 271

sprint workout, 300-301

Squat(s), 34, 46, 204, 229, 268

    with band, 76

    Body-Weight, 91, 311

    Box, 270

    Bulgarian Split, 28, 58, 87, 213, 226, 231, 271

    Bulgarian Split Squat Iso Hold, 211

    Dumbbell, 59, 203

    Front, 30, 53, 240

    Front Squat to Press, 41

Jump, 94, 205, 208
　Overhead, 15
　Pause, 200
　Prisoner, 326
　Skater, 210
　Split Squat to Press, 50
　Sumo, 292
　Sumo Squat Hold, 22
　Touch-Touch, 21
　Wall, 233
stairclimbers, 273
　workout for, 284
Staley, Charles, 316
Standing Calf Raise, 37, 216
Standing Dumbbell Flye, 167
Starnes, Shelby, 6
Star Plank, 251
Stepup, 57, 59, 100, 101, 325
　Dumbbell, 202
Straight-Leg Barbell Situp, 241
strength training:
　medicine-ball workouts as useful for, 84
　warmup exercises for, 19-20
　see also workouts; specific exercises
stretches, 14-18, 105, 160, 179, 180, 227, 240
Suitcase Deadlift, 241
Sumo Romanian Deadlift, 228
Sumo Squat, 292
Sumo Squat Hold, 22
Superman, 193
suspension-trainer workouts:
　for arms, 108-9
　for back, 196-97
　for butt, 230-31
　for chest, 154-57
　full-body, 79-81
　for legs, 212-13
　for shoulders, 176-77
swimming workout, 294
Swiss Ball Plank, 40
Swiss Ball Rollout, 29
Swiss-ball workouts:
　for abs, 248-49

　for butt, 232-33
　full-body, 89-91

T
Tabata, Izumi, 328
Tap Out, 81
Tate Press, 128, 130
tempo, in workouts, 27
testosterone, 8, 10, 186
30-minute workout, 316-17
3-Way Finisher, 157
3-Way Flye, 154
3-Way Shoulder Finisher, 197
thrusts, 232, 234
　Barbell Hip, 224
　Butterfly Hip, 233
　Feet-On-Ball Hip, 232
　Frog, 292
Tiptoe Walk, 221
Toe Touch, 247
Toe-Touch Squat, 21
T on Ball, 90
Towel Cable Row, 138
Towel Curl, 142
Towel Kettlebell Curl, 139
Towel Pullup, 139
Towel Row to Chest, 139
Trap-Bar Deadlift, 38
Trap Raise, 169
traps, exercises for, 253-57
　barbell-only, 254-55
　dumbbell-only, 256-57
treadmills, 273, 274, 318
　workout for, 276
triceps, exercises for, 33, 34-35, 39, 77, 105, 106, 108-9, 111, 123-35, 158, 162
　band-only, 132-33
　barbell-only, 126-27
　body-weight, 134-35
　dumbell-only, 128-31
　full-gym, 124-25
　in short workouts, 317
Triceps Extension, 109, 111, 133, 135, 163
　Decline, 125

Decline EZ-Bar, 33
Decline EZ-Bar Lying, 39
Double-Band, 133
Lying, 127, 129
Neutral-Grip, 105
Pullover, 106
Triceps Pushdown, 77
triset muscles, 178
TRX, 79, 80
Turkish Getup, 64
20-minute workouts, 318-25
Two-Dumbbell/Kettlebell Workout, 56-65

U
Underhand Kickback, 130
Uni-Bridge Press, 81
upper-body workouts, 259-65
USDA Food Pyramid, 5
USDA MyPlate, 6

V
vegetables, 9
versaclimber workout, 286
V-Up, 246
and Pass, 249

W
Walking Lunge, 201, 269
1.5, 211
Walking Single-Leg Romanian Deadlift, 225
Wall Ankle Mobilization, 240
Wall Squat, 233
warmup exercises, 13-23
for strength training, 19-20
Weighted Back Extension, 271
Weighted Pullup, 35
Weighted Situp, 269
Wide-Grip Curl, 117
Wide-Grip Pullup, 194
Wide-Grip Pushup, 161
"working up," 19-20
workouts:
band-only, 73-77, 107, 120-21, 132-33, 160-61, 172-75, 242-43

barbell-only, 49-53, 106, 116-17, 126-27, 142-43, 150-51, 188-89, 204-7, 226-29, 240-41, 254-55
for body recomposition, 26-33
body-weight, 93-101, 134-35, 162-63, 178-81, 194-95, 208-11, 234-35, 250-51
cardio, see cardio workouts
dropsets in, 194, 262
dumbbell/kettlebell-only, 55-65, 104-5, 118-19, 128-31, 140-41, 152-53, 182-83, 190-93, 202-3, 218-19, 256-57
full-body, see full-body workouts
full-gym, 25-47, 114-15, 124-25, 138-39, 146-49, 166-69, 186-87, 200-201, 216-17, 224-25, 238-39
lower-body, 267-71
machine, 67-71, 273-87
medicine ball, 83-87, 246-47
nutrition for, 10
performing reps in, 56, 68, 94, 98, 104, 116, 118, 120, 132, 134, 150, 158, 162, 166, 186, 196, 216, 246, 250, 262, 268
short, see short workouts
for specific body parts, see body-part workouts
speed work in, 150
suspension-trainer, 79-81, 108-9, 154-57, 176-77, 196-97, 212-13, 230-31
Swiss-ball, 89-91, 232-33, 248-49
tempo in, 27
upper-body, 259-65
warmups to, 13-23
W Raise, 175
Wrist Curl, 141
Reverse, 141
wrist straps, 137

Y
Yates Row, 189
Y Raise, 177
Y to W Raise, 179

Z
Zinczenko, David, xiii-xv
Zottman Curl, 265
Seated, 32